G000123736

Cognitive Behavioral Therapy

A Simple CBT Guide to Overcoming Anxiety, Intrusive Thoughts, Worry and Depression along with Tips for Using Mindfulness to Rewire Your Brain

© **Copyright 2019 - All rights reserved.**

The contents of this book may not be reproduced, duplicated, or transmitted without direct written permission from the author.

Under no circumstances will any legal responsibility or blame be held against the publisher for any reparation, damages, or monetary loss due to the information herein, either directly or indirectly.

Legal Notice:

This book is copyright protected. This is only for personal use. You cannot amend, distribute, sell, use, quote, or paraphrase any part of the content within this book without the consent of the author.

Disclaimer Notice:

Please note the information contained within this document is for educational and entertainment purposes only. Every attempt has been made to provide accurate, up to date, and reliable information. No warranties of any kind are expressed or implied. Readers acknowledge that the author is not engaging in the rendering of legal, financial, medical, or professional advice. The content of this book has been derived from various sources. Please consult a licensed professional before attempting any techniques outlined in this book.

By reading this document, the reader agrees that under no circumstances is the author or publisher responsible for any losses, direct or indirect, which are incurred as a result of the use of the information contained within this document, including, but not limited to errors, omissions, or inaccuracies. Any icons used in this book are the property of Freepik and received through a Basic License. Besides, files from the Wikimedia Commons are used. Commons is a freely licensed media file repository. All credit belongs to the authors/creators.

Contents

Introduction

Cognitive-behavioral therapy (CBT) has become one of the best methods of psychotherapy for treating several mental health problems. Although it is a relatively new method of treatment, it has gained popularity among many experts around the world. It is important to note that CBT doesn't take away problems; instead, it helps people with mild to severe mental illness to cope and deal with their issues more effectively.

This method of psychotherapy is based on changing and modifying the way you behave. This book aims to create an awareness of CBT, going in-depth to provide you with the mechanisms of action and showing you the inner workings of what CBT is all about.

One of the things discussed is the history of CBT, which will provide you with valid information while you explore the various steps involved in CBT development.

Another essential factor explored is the role of negative thoughts in mental health. What we think about a particular situation affects how we see it, perceive it, how we respond to it, and our behavior towards it. We'll explore the origin of negative thoughts and how a specific pattern of thinking affects our reactions and responses.

Also, we get to see what a typical CBT session looks like and the role of the therapist in helping people with mental health problems. CBT is a therapy that depends on a particular structure; it differs from other treatments in the construction of and the amount of time needed for the procedure. Also, an essential factor differentiating CBT from other methods of psychotherapy is the relationship between the therapist and the patient.

CBT is a goal-oriented therapy, so it is best suited for mental health issues that can be broken down into goals.

Identification of mental health problems is critical, as it helps you to deal with them faster and with better results. Recognition of various health disorders such as depression, anxiety, schizophrenia, panic attacks, excessive worrying, and other mental health illnesses is achieved through observation of the various symptoms. Being able to pinpoint the symptoms of these mental health problems is the first step towards treatment. Many of these mental health problems have similar signs and symptoms, so it is essential to seek the help of an expert to recognize the particular health problem you might be facing.

Goal setting is an essential and fundamental part of CBT. We cannot overemphasize the importance of goal setting because this is one of the first requirements in CBT treatment. Goal setting in CBT has a mechanism that is achieved only by following the correct approach. You will learn how to set realistic and achievable goals in Chapter Three.

Anxiety and worry are prevalent mental health issues around the world. CBT treatment for anxiety and stress consists of asking the right questions and being able to assess yourself correctly. With the help of CBT, you will be able to identify negative thought patterns that often lead to anxiety and worry and to challenge them by replacing them with more realistic ones. In the treatment of anxiety and stress disorders, you and your therapist will work together to come up with various assignments or homework which will help you to apply everything learned in the therapy sessions.

Depression is another major mental health illness that affects many people in this day and age. It is now a common feature of modern-day life and is poised to become one of the most common health problems of our time. There are various types of depression, and identifying the type that you may be experiencing requires professional assistance. CBT treatment for depression often follows the typical goal-oriented, structured plan that is characteristic of CBT. Unlike other psychotherapy for depression, CBT offers a shorter therapy time, with less chance of relapse. The various tools and techniques derived from CBT sessions can be used long after you've completed the therapy sessions. The treatments remain viable and applicable throughout your life and reduce the risk of relapse.

The relationship between substance abuse and depression is a common topic when it comes to mental illness. Many people who have depression are susceptible to developing addiction problems; this diagnosis is referred to as a dual diagnosis.

Work-related stress is a significant concern, as an increasing number of workers are now experiencing work-related stress at an alarming rate. Because of the growing pressure to achieve more in less time, many people often end up feeling as though they have underachieved, which serves as a significant source of work-related stress. We provide information on the triggers, symptoms, and long-term effect of workplace stress. CBT treatment for workplace stress has been effective in helping many people come up with different strategies for managing it efficiently. CBT helps you to come up with a realistic plan to deal with stressful situations at work by helping you prioritize, keep track of your moods, and feel less overwhelmed at work.

Intrusive thoughts are the leading cause of many mental health problems such as anxiety, depression, Obsessive-Compulsive Disorder (OCD), and others. CBT treatment for intrusive thoughts will help you to identify these thoughts and the triggers responsible for them.

The relationship between CBT and mindfulness is discussed in great detail. The histories and similarities between mindfulness and CBT will help you to understand their usefulness in tackling many mental health issues.

The combination of CBT and mindfulness has produced results that make MBCT an invaluable tool in dealing with mental health problems such as depression and anxiety. MBCT applies the principles of both CBT and mindfulness. If you are tired of various other methods of treatments that just haven't worked for you and you're looking for something more refreshing with a higher rate of success, then CBT might be for you.

Chapter One: Why Use CBT?

Cognitive-behavioral therapy (CBT) aims to improve your general mental and emotional state with the use of a practical approach. It helps you understand complex and challenging cognitive distortions in your thoughts, feelings, and attitudes to improve the ability to function and the overall quality of life. It was designed initially to treat depression and other mental illnesses, but it is now being applied extensively in the treatment of various psychogenic problems ranging from sleep disorders to drug and alcohol abuse, depression, severe mental illness, eating disorders, and anxiety. By paying attention to beliefs, attitude, and lifestyles, it aids you in identifying thinking patterns responsible for ineffective behavior and negative moods. Identifying these patterns improves your emotional control and helps you to develop coping strategies against emotional difficulties that lead to depression.

CBT also features an essential advantage over several other treatment methods; it is a short-term treatment compared to others. For most emotional problems it has a treatment plan ranging between five to ten months. It features a smaller amount of sessions per week, each lasting for approximately 60 minutes. During the sessions, you work with the therapist to identify the psychological triggers that impede typical day to day function. Throughout the therapy sessions the therapist introduces several techniques that can be applied when the need arises, and these principles can be used over a lifetime.

CBT is based on the principle of the addition of behavioral therapy to psychotherapy. Behavioral therapy focuses on the role our problems play in affecting our thoughts, behavior, and general lifestyle. Psychotherapy pays close attention to the beginning of our thinking pattern in childhood and how the importance we place on things affects our response to them. It then aids people in challenging those automatic thoughts, reactions, or beliefs that come when triggered by specific situations, using appropriate strategies to modify their behavior to more positive responses and thought.

The History of Cognitive Behavioral Therapy

Aaron Beck is credited for inventing Cognitive Behavioral Therapy in 1960. He was a psychoanalyst, and while in analytical sessions he saw that his patients had conversations with themselves, similar to those between two people. But his patients never gave a full report of their thoughts.

For instance, during a session of therapy, you might be thinking to yourself, "He (the therapist) doesn't understand anything I'm saying," and you might end up feeling annoyed or displeased as a result of this thought. Consequently, you could respond to the previous thought with another one: "Maybe it's my fault for not being forthcoming with what I feel." The next thought might end up changing how you felt previously due to the first thought.

Aaron finally came to recognize the importance of the relationship between feelings and thoughts. He then coined the term "*Automatic Thought*" to explain emotion-filled ideas that come up from time to time in our minds. He concluded that people are not always aware of these thoughts but can still be taught to identify and report them. He concluded that the key to someone dealing with such difficulties is recognizing and understanding the roles these thoughts play on their emotions and behavior.

Because of the importance of the relationship between thoughts and behavior, Aaron came up with the term *"Cognitive Therapy"* for this method of psychology. Today, it is recognized as Cognitive-behavioral therapy (CBT). The balance between psychotherapy and behavioral treatment can be adjusted to suit individual needs; this has led to the founding of many categories of CBT. CBT has undergone several scientific trials by various teams, and its range of applications has increased through the years.

The Role of Negative Thoughts

The theory supporting CBT is that events alone are not what is responsible for what we feel or how we behave, but also the meaning and importance we place on them. For example, if one experiences a barrage of negative thoughts it could distort their perception and lead them into believing what is not so. They may cling to this distorted set of thoughts and beliefs and fail to accept anything to the contrary.

For instance, due to depression, a student might think, "I'm incapable of getting through school today because nothing will go right; everyone hates me, I have no friends, and I will be all alone." As a result of believing this thought, they might claim to be sick to avoid going to school. By responding and letting this thought affect his or her behavior, he or she takes away the chance of discovering if her prediction is going to be wrong. If the student had ignored this thought and took the opportunity of going to school, something might have been different, or things might have gone better than their prediction. But they choose to stay at home, dealing with even more negative thoughts like, "I've missed a lot today, and I'm so lonely." Views like this could lead to the student feeling even worse and reduce the chances of them going to school the next day. Situations like these are the beginning of a downward spiral. Vicious circles like these often apply to many other problems.

Where Do These Negative Thoughts Come From?

According to Aaron, every individual establishes their thinking pattern during childhood, and they go on to create a reflexive or automatic way of thinking that remains fixed. For instance, consider a situation where the parents generally neglected their child (except in times of need), but the child does well in school. In this instance, the child will end up thinking, "I have to be at the top of my game in school, so I do well, or else my parents will reject me." The child ends up coming up with a rule for his/her existence (referred to as dysfunctional assumption). This rule might be distorted, but it might also enable the child to work harder to do well in school so as to gain more attention from their parents.

This pattern leads to several trains of thought known as dysfunctional thought patterns, which are activated or triggered when something beyond the control of the child happens. When this occurs, the established automatic model of thoughts takes center stage in the child's mind, precipitating thoughts such as, "I am a failure and have no reason for existence."

The role of cognitive-behavioral therapy is to help people in similar situations to understand what is happening. It helps them think outside their established reflexive lines of thought. So, in the case of the student who is worried about how alone they would feel in class, CBT encourages and aids them to examine real-life situations and see what happens. When the student takes the chance and puts themselves in a more realistic real-life state, they might experience things that would go better than they had expected; they may meet someone who shares the same life-view and make a friend for a change, so that they can feel less lonely.

It is an absolute fact that things don't always go as planned. Still, when your mind is unstable, your thoughts, predictions, and interpretations will be distorted; you don't see things clearly, and you will have greater difficulty dealing with worse situations. CBT helps you correct distorted views and interpretations you might have of various circumstances.

What is CBT Treatment Like? What to Expect in CBT Sessions

CBT is different from other types of therapy in some essential ways. If you are considering CBT as a course of treatment, it might help to have an idea of what to expect in CBT sessions.

CBT Sessions

In the first session, the primary purpose is to come up with an assessment of the situation. The meeting allows you to explain in detail the problems you are experiencing. In this session, the therapist will try to get a full picture of the essential factors needed in the care. The therapist then determines if they are the right fit for you in helping you deal with your problems, or if they need to refer you to someone else. At the end of the first session, the therapist is usually able to come up with a treatment plan listing various interventions needed for the therapy. In some cases, it takes more than one session to create a comprehensive treatment plan. After crafting the schedule, the therapist helps you understand if the treatment plan is perfect for you.

After the assessment, treatment begins in subsequent sessions to deal with the objective of the treatment plan. In each session, time is given to solving problems, in contrast to the traditional treatment that involves a lot of talking about the problems.

At every session, CBT maximizes the use of time for greater effectiveness. Every session starts with a little check-in to determine how effective the treatment plan is in solving the underlying problem. A quick recap of the last session and homework follows this check-in. After going through this, the rest of the meeting is spent dealing with the agenda of the day.

Concluding Sessions

When you've met the goal(s) of the treatment plan, the therapist reduces the frequency of the sessions. Other conventional therapy sometimes lasts for three years. However, CBT lasts for just a few months. The reason is that the CBT design aims to make you your own therapist by providing you with the tools to cope with any situation. Therapists schedule the last phase of CBT sessions less frequently, giving you more time to apply the skills and tools you have learned to real-life situations and to build up your confidence in your ability to deal with subsequent problems that may arise.

At the end of each session, the therapist often gives homework; this is a vital process as it helps people master the tools or skills acquired during the sessions. Homework varies depending on the nature of the agenda of a particular therapy session. For instance, you might be asked to keep records of incidents that trigger emotions of depression or anxiety. This assignment might be imperative to examining the thoughts generated due to the events. The next task could be to apply specific skills learned during the therapy sessions to deal with similar situations.

How CBT Differs from Other Therapies

The significant difference between CBT and other therapies lies in the relationship between you and the therapist. An innate drawback of most treatments is that they might create a sort of dependency on the therapist. As a result, you might come to view the therapist as all-powerful and all-knowing. With CBT, this is not the case.

In CBT, the relationship between you and the therapist is more or less an equal one, more like a business arrangement, more practical and problem-focused. Your therapist always asks questions on your views about the therapy. Aaron Beck described this relationship with the term "*Collaborative Empiricism*". It stresses the importance of you working together with the therapist in coming up with ideas to apply to your issues.

Benefits of Cognitive-Behavioral Therapy

The National Association of Cognitive-Behavioral Therapists (NACBT) have described the foundation of CBT as being built on the theory that our behavior and feelings occur in response to our thoughts, and they are not caused by things like situations, people, and events. With this fact, the advantage is that we can alter our views to change our feelings and act contrary to a case or circumstance.

Benefits of CBT include

- Ability to identify negative emotions and thoughts
- In cases of addiction, deterring relapse
- Help in anger management
- Coping with grief and loss
- Managing chronic pain
- Overcoming trauma and dealing with PTSD
- Overcoming sleep disorders
- Resolving relationship difficulties

Who Can Benefit from CBT Treatment?

CBT is often a suitable treatment for people with specific problems; for people who are just experiencing feelings of unhappiness and unfulfillment but lack the symptoms that prevent them from getting through everyday life, CBT may be less helpful.

CBT is useful for the following problems

- Anxiety and panic attacks
- Intrusive thoughts
- Depression

- Worrying

- Anger management

- Child and adolescent problems

- Chronic fatigue syndrome

- Chronic pain

- Mood swings

- Habits, such as facial tics

- Eating Disorders

- Obsessive-compulsive disorder (OCD)

- General health problems

- Drug or alcohol addiction

- Phobias

- Sleep disorders

- Sexual and relationship issues

- Post-traumatic stress disorder (PTSD)

Mindfulness-Based Cognitive Therapy (MBCT)

Founded by Zindel Segal, Mark Williams, and John Teasdale, MBCT was designed initially to deal with depression, but it is now applicable to a wide range of problems.

MBCT is a psychological treatment that combines techniques of cognitive-behavioral therapy (CBT) with strategies of mindfulness to help individuals better understand and manage their emotions and thoughts. MBCT generally helps individuals achieve alleviation from feelings of distress.

Chapter Two: Identifying Mental Health Disorders

The World Health Organization has given us a clear definition of good mental health; it says that it is a state of well-being where an individual realizes their abilities, can work productively, can deal with the regular, day-to-day stress of life, and can contribute to his or her community.

Mental health disorders include a wide range of various problems, with different signs and symptoms but are characterized by a combination of abnormal emotions, behavior, thoughts, and relationships. Instances of mental health disorders are depression, schizophrenia, intellectual disabilities, and complications due to drug abuse and anxiety disorders. Most of these disorders can be successfully treated.

Mental health disorders can affect relationships, daily life, and sometimes physical health. According to experts, everyone has the potential to develop mental health disorders, regardless of age, ethnic group, gender, or financial status.

Cognitive-behavioral therapy (CBT) used either alone or together with other treatments has been applied to treating several mental health disorders. Besides treating mental health problems, CBT can be used to deal with stress.

We are going to focus on identifying some of the most common mental health disorders, such as anxiety disorders, worry and depression, mood disorders, and schizophrenia.

Anxiety Disorders

Anxiety disorder occurs as a result of extreme fear or anxiety, which can be triggered by specific situations, sounds, and objects. Individuals with this disorder try to keep away from the triggers of their distress.

Some anxiety disorders include:

Panic Disorder

This disorder occurs when you experience sudden paralyzing terror or have a sense of impending disaster.

Phobias

These range from simple phobias such as social phobias (fear of being judged by others) to agoraphobia (fear of being unable to get out of certain situations) to disproportionate dread of objects.

Obsessive-Compulsive Disorder (OCD)

OCD is an anxiety disorder characterized by a feeling of intense urgency, compulsions, and obsessions. For instance, having an intense urge to wash your hand repetitively.

Post-Traumatic Stress Disorder (PTSD)

PTSD occurs in the aftermath of a traumatic event when someone experience or witness something frightening and horrible. During this event, you may have felt threatened or that you had no control over what was happening.

Some signs and symptoms of anxiety include:

Excessive Worrying

One of the most common symptoms of an anxiety disorder is worrying. This emotion is normal in people, but here, the amount of fear in a situation is distorted or not proportionate to the trigger. This symptom is a sign of anxiety disorder if it continues for six months or more and the worry becomes difficult to control, interferes with your daily tasks, and makes it hard to concentrate.

Feeling Agitated

The feeling of anxiousness causes overstimulation of the nervous system which results in a series of connected events that occur throughout the body, such as sweaty palms, a racing pulse, dry mouth, and shaky hands. All these symptoms occur when the body believes it is in immediate danger, so the nervous system prepares the body for it. Blood is diverted away from the gastrointestinal tract to your muscles in preparation for the reaction of fight or flight. Your heart rate increases, and all your senses are alert. These changes are necessary to keep you safe in times of actual danger, but in the case of anxiety disorders, the threat is all in your head. People with anxiety disorder often have a hard time calming their feelings of agitation.

Panic Attacks

A primary symptom of anxiety disorder is a panic attack. This symptom manifests as an overwhelming and intense feeling of fright.

Following the panic attack is an increase in the heart rate, shortness of breath, shaking, tightness of the chest, nausea, sweating, and loss of control. If panic attacks occur frequently, then it may be a sign of anxiety disorder.

Trouble Falling or Staying Asleep

Sleep disorders usually accompany anxiety disorders. You might have a hard time falling asleep and/or staying asleep. According to some studies, children who have insomnia are more at risk of developing an anxiety disorder later in life. This symptom is strongly related to anxiety, and treatment of anxiety disorders improves sleep as well.

Restlessness

Restlessness is a common sign of anxiety disorder, especially in teens and children. People with this symptom tend to be on edge and have an uncontrollable urge to move. This symptom might not occur in everyone with anxiety, but it is an essential symptom of anxiety disorders. Experiencing restlessness for more than six months is a sign of an anxiety disorder.

Irrational Fears

Intense fear of certain things such as enclosed spaces, heights, and spiders could be a sign of phobia. Phobia is the irrational fear of a particular situation or object. This fear impairs your ability to carry out everyday functions.

Common Phobias Include

- Phobia of animals
- Situational phobias
- Phobia of the natural environment
- Phobia of blood/injections/injury
- Avoiding social situations

You might be displaying indications of social anxiety disorder if you find yourself having a fear of social events, fear of being judged or examined by others, or the fear of public humiliation.

Avoiding Social Situations

Social anxiety is common, even among adults, at some point in their lives. It is commonly developed during childhood and is usually common in early teens. An individual with this symptom tends to appear extremely quiet and shy when meeting new people or in group settings; though they may hide this on the outside, on the inside they have extreme fear and distress. Some people can appear standoffish or snobby as be a result of high self-criticism, depression, or low self-esteem.

Difficulty Concentrating

People with anxiety disorders often have a hard time concentrating. According to some studies anxiety impairs working memory, making it impossible to hold on to short term memories. However, it's important to note that not being able to concentrate is a sign of other disorders as well, such as depression, so it not an exclusive symptom of anxiety disorder.

Depression

Feelings of unhappiness are different from that of depression. Depression is a mental health disorder that is more complicated. It is a significant mental health disorder that leads to difficulty in carrying out simple daily tasks.

Feelings of sadness are part of our everyday life. Still, when you start to experience emotions like despair and hopelessness that won't go away, you risk a downward spiral into depression.

It is essential to take note of the signs and symptoms that point towards depression to determine if they are the natural feelings of sadness that most people tend to sometimes go through in life.

Hopeless Outlook

A primary symptom of depression is the way people with this disorder perceive life. They have a pessimistic or helpless view of life which prevents them from functioning. They may also have feelings of worthlessness, self-hate, and intense guilt, believing everything is their fault.

Loss of Interest

People with depression often cannot feel pleasure or enjoy things. They experience a loss of interest in everything in general, even those things they once loved. Loss of sex drive and/or impotence are primarily associated with depression.

Increased Fatigue and Sleep Problems

As a result of the inability to enjoy the things you love, you feel a never-ending sense of fatigue. You might feel a lack of energy or have an excessive urge to sleep. Depression can also be associated with insomnia.

Anxiety

Depression and anxiety can occur simultaneously, and often go hand in hand. It is essential to note that not all forms of anxiety are symptoms of depression. Some things that can be associated with anxiety include:

- Feelings of dread

- Fast and increased heart rate

- Nervous breathing

- Restlessness and tension

- Overthinking and lack of focus

- Increased sweating

These symptoms can be managed with CBT.

Irritability in Men

Depression tends to be different for men and women. Depressed men usually have characteristic behaviors such as irritation, substance abuse, and misplaced anger. Unlike women, men with depression find it difficult to recognize depression and seek treatment.

Changes in Appetite and Weight

Weight fluctuation is one of the primary characteristics of depression, and it is different from one individual to another. In some, it leads to a gain in weight, while in others, it can lead to weight loss. Depression is known to affect appetite, and it can differ from one person to the next as to whether it pushes them to overeat or not eat at all.

Uncontrollable Emotions

When depressed, you might get periodic outbursts of anger. Your feelings can be all over the place; you can go from feeling an intense amount of anger from the smallest trigger at one moment, and the next you may find yourself wallowing in self-pity or crying for no apparent reason.

Looking at Death

The leading cause of suicide is depression. A large number of people die each year as a result of depression that has gone untreated. They often see it as a way out of their problems because, from their point of view, there's no other way out. They may talk about how they often consider taking their own lives. If you think someone is at risk of committing suicide as a result of depression, it is crucial to get them help as soon as possible.

Mood Disorders

This mental health disorder is primarily concerned with the emotional state of a person. The person experiences extremes of highs and lows, of happiness and sadness, or sometimes even both.

Humans have the natural ability to alter their moods on the basis of their surrounding environment. However, in the case of mood disorder, the ability to handle routine or normal daily activities is interrupted and challenging.

Common symptoms of mood disorders include:

- Feeling sad almost all the time or nearly every day

- Feeling worthless or hopeless

- Lack of energy or feeling sluggish

- Gaining weight or losing weight

- Extremes of appetite (high or low)

- Lack of sleep or oversleeping

- No interest in activities that you normally enjoy

- Frequent thoughts about death or suicide

- Difficulty concentrating or focusing

- High-level energy

- Fast speech or movement

- Perturbation, unease, or touchiness

- Risk-taking behavior such as driving recklessly or drinking excessively

- An abnormal increase in activity or an atypical urge do too many things at once

- Contending thoughts

- Feeling apprehensive or edgy for no apparent reason

Schizophrenia

Schizophrenia is a serious and debilitating mental disorder wherein people have a distorted view of reality. It is usually characterized by hallucinations, resulting in the inability to carry out daily functions. Schizophrenia requires lifelong treatments to manage. In the early stages, medical care is given to manage the symptoms and improve lifestyle.

Features of this mental health disorder involve a range of emotional and behavioral problems, and the inability to distinguish the difference between what is real and what isn't. Common signs and symptoms vary from person to person. Symptoms like speech impairment, hallucinations, and delusions cause great difficulty in functioning effectively.

Symptoms of schizophrenia include:

Delusions

People with schizophrenia have difficulty in perceiving reality, as some of their beliefs are false and are not based upon reality as most people see it. For instance, people with schizophrenia may believe that they are being harmed and harassed, that there is a significant disaster coming, that someone is in love with them, that they have attained exceptional fame, or that they have gotten a dream job. Most people with schizophrenia have these kinds of delusions.

Hallucinations

Hallucinations are another significant sign of schizophrenia. It involves hearing and seeing things that are not there. This symptom could occur in any of the senses, but the most common is the patient hearing voices in their head. The next is seeing things that aren't there.

Disorganized Thoughts (speech)

Schizophrenia is also characterized by uncoordinated expression as a result of disordered thinking. This makes it challenging to communicate and pass information. "Word salad" is the term used to describe the situation where they utter meaningless words as they attempt to express themselves.

Extremely Disorganized or Abnormal Motor Behavior

People with schizophrenia also may exhibit childlike silliness and compulsive agitation. They find it hard to accomplish tasks as they lose track of the goal or purpose of a given job. Other common behaviors include resistance to instructions, strange postures, excessive and unproductive movements, and refusal to respond while being talked to.

Negative Symptoms

This symptom is characterized by the inability to function properly. For instance, appearing emotionless (failing to make eye contact, having no facial expression, and talking in a monotone). People with this condition experience a loss of interest in various activities, social withdrawal, and an inability to feel pleasure.

Over time the person experiences periods of heightened symptoms and periods of remission; however, some symptoms may persist regularly.

For men, studies show that schizophrenia usually begins between their early to mid-twenties, while for women, it usually starts in the late twenties. Schizophrenia is rare in children and for individuals above the age of 45.

Symptoms in Teenagers

Though the symptoms of schizophrenia are the same in adults and teenagers, the symptoms are more difficult to recognize in children. This is because early symptoms are similar to the expected behavior of teens in general, so schizophrenia in teens can go unnoticed for some time. Some of these symptoms include:

- Keeping a distance from friends and family

- Reduced performance in school

- Sleeping disturbance

- Bad mood

- A feeling of doing nothing

Compared to schizophrenic adults, teens are less likely to have delusions and more likely to have visual hallucinations.

Severe symptoms like extreme shock, loss of control, loss of touch with reality, hallucinations, urge to self-harm, and suicidal thoughts in mental health disorders are considered psychological red flags. If by chance, you notice any of these symptoms, you must seek professional advice immediately.

Chapter Three: Goal Setting: Your Starting Point to Mental and Emotional Wellness

The CBT method has its foundation based on the collaboration between you and the therapist to design strategies and structure to maintain focus. In other words, CBT is designed to be goal oriented. The whole point is to make the reason for the therapy relevant to you. The goal is emphasized by the therapist to give you a clear view of what you want instead of what you think you want.

The Therapeutic Relationship in CBT

In CBT, the collaborative relationship between you and the therapist is important; it is referred to as a "therapeutic relationship". In this relationship, the therapist acts more like a mentor or guide as opposed to the instructor in other types of therapies where you are told what to do. In CBT, the therapist acts in a supporting role, pushing and encouraging you towards exploring new options on how to control your thought process to manage your behavior and feelings. This relationship plays a vital role as you work with the therapist to come up with realistic goals to determine what you hope to accomplish.

How Goals Work

Creating goals helps you to focus on what is relevant and essential. It also helps you develop a vision of the place you want to be in your life, or how you would ideally want your life to be. Setting a goal increases your effort or decreases your energy on specific activities to help you come up with strategies to achieve the goal.

Generally, goal setting in mental health is an essential step used to recover from any common mental health problems such as anxiety and depression. Cognitive Behavior therapy is the first step in overcoming such issues.

Approach to Goals

There are many different ways or paths to goal setting. In CBT, the "S.M.A.R.T." way is one of the most used strategies. This method gives you a vivid and clear picture of your goal or what you hope to accomplish. It aids you in maintaining your zeal or motivation for achieving your purpose. Below is the full meaning of the acronym "S.M.A.R.T."

S-Specific

Being specific means that your goal is clear and focused on what you want. This ensures that you avoid generalization and increases the chances of accomplishing your desired goal.

M-Measurable

Being a measurable goal enables you to quantitatively and qualitatively create margins for what you want. It gives you a concrete criterion toward achieving each goal set. You need to ask yourself, "How many?" and "How much?", and, "How will I know when my goal has been attained?"

A-Achievable

Your goals need to be achievable and feasible. Questions like, "How are you going to go about achieving your goals?" and "What can you do to make meeting your goals possible?" need to be asked.

R-Realistic

This is one of the most important aspects of goal setting. Your goals need to be within the limit of what you think you can do within the time frame you have given yourself. Is the goal achievable given your current circumstances? Though setting big goals can serve to motivate you towards working hard, it can be disappointing when they are not achieved because they are set too far beyond your capabilities. This can leave you feeling even worse.

T-Timely

The time frame for achieving each goal must be within a realistic limit. This helps you to avoid procrastination that could lead to you giving up on your goals.

Below are two examples of achieving your goals with this approach in CBT.

A person not currently exercising has the desire to exercise frequently. What they might be able to put together using the SMART approach is:

S-Specific: Every 20 minutes, I will jog around the nearby park.

M-Measurable: I will keep a diary or record the number of times I go jogging and for how long.

A-Achievable: I will ask a friend to join me on each jog so that I am obligated to go out.

R-Realistic: 20 minutes is more than enough time to have a good morning jog around the park, so it is enough to get my juices flowing, and with my friend with me the run will be super fun.

T-Timely: I will keep up this routine for a month, and after that I will have a review of how much success I have had in achieving this goal.

The second example is Michael, who experiences panic attacks as a result of severe anxiety. Michael's academics are greatly affected as a result of the stress, even though he is a good student. He finally gets through college and begins work, and now deals with anxiety and occasional panic attacks when interacting with his colleagues. He decides to set the goal of coming up with a way of dealing with the anxiety disorder to improve his mental health. Applying the smart method, this is what he can come up with:

S-Specific: he has concluded that he needs to reduce his anxious feelings and to decrease his panic attacks.

M-Measurable: to make his goal more measurable, he decides to keep a daily record of his moods and grade the level of his anxiety on a scale of 1-10. He will do this each time he experiences the slightest hint of a panic attack. This is so he can get the data he needs to determine if there is any change with time.

A-Achievable: the goal of becoming less anxious and more confident is one that many people have achieved, so it is a pretty easy goal to achieve.

Realistic: the goal is a realistic one that is within the limits of his power. After seeking help and gathering the necessary information needed via the Internet and other means of research, he confirmed that his goal is achievable. He found a therapist and was advised that though his goal is possible, it requires a lot of personal hard work, but he can reduce the rate and level of anxiety he feels to manageable levels.

T-Time

With the daily record-keeping he hopes to see noticeable changes by the time he analyses his data after a year and a half. At that time, he hopes to feel more confident in dealing with more challenges at the workplace.

In these examples, both people were able to come up with a well-thought-out goal backed up with a plan that was both realistic and within achievable limits. In time, both goals have a high chance of becoming reality. The S.M.A.R.T. approach provides you with a step-by-step plan that provides the most comfortable possible route toward achieving your goal.

Role of Homework in Achieving Your Goals

As mentioned in Chapter One, homework is an essential aspect of CBT. It is following the strategy and plan set out to make your goal a reality. If you want to get better and improve your mental health, this part of CBT is a must.

The activities or assignments will depend mainly on the therapeutic relationship between you and the therapist. After every session, you and the therapist come up with jobs that will provide you with opportunities to put what you have gained so far in the sessions into practice. The therapy itself is an excellent setting to gain useful insight that you may not have been able to see without guidance. So basically, the purpose of these assignments is for you to align and put the things you've learned into practice. This helps you gain real-life experiences and come to an understanding of just how much better you can become at controlling your thoughts and behaviors.

In addition to doing these assignments between sessions, you will also have to keep a record of your findings on the CBT worksheet.

An example of an assignment is keeping records of your thoughts in response to certain different situations to help you identify those objects, things, locations that serve as triggers for specific unhealthy thought processes.

Steps in Achieving your Goals

Breaking Down Goals

If your goal consists of many working parts, then breaking it into smaller segments is not a bad idea. It allows you to have a sense of accomplishment that maintains your focus, and therefore, you don't have to feel overwhelmed.

Sometimes the goals of people with a mental health problem are ambiguous and unspecific, such as:

· I want to feel happier

· I want to feel better about myself and gain self-confidence

· I need to stop being anxious all the time and become more relaxed

All these goals are ambitious, and there is nothing wrong with them. However, they are not specific enough. They are too broad because you don't know where to start; what do you do, how do you accomplish it, and how do you know how far you have gone in achieving the goal? These are questions you need to ask yourself.

To help you to establish a reasonable and realistic goal, below are a few steps to help you to break down your goal into smaller achievable goals.

The first step is asking yourself - how do you want to live your life once accomplishing the goal?

With this question, you move a step closer to achieving your desired state of mind, even though it doesn't do much to rid you of anxiety, low self-esteem, or depression. Some questions you can ask yourself at this stage are:

· What do you want to experience to feel better about yourself?

· What statements would you begin to make when you have succeeded in increasing your self-confidence?

29

· What engagements will you have with your increased self-confidence? What will be your approach to life?

The next step is for you to find real answers to your questions.

You will have to recognize specific thoughts and behaviors as guides. Below are some probable answers:

-With me being happier, I can spend more time with my friends and colleagues. I will have at least three social outings with them as a sign of me feeling more satisfied.

-When talking to myself, I will congratulate myself on handling certain situations. I will feel proud of myself for having those social outings and for being happier.

Set a Time Frame for Achieving Your Goals

You will need to keep track and record your progress on a daily or weekly basis. You will have to keep track of how many times time you go out with your friends and how many times you congratulate yourself on a job well done, as well as record things that prevented you from achieving your goals.

The routine check enables you to see your progress and gauge how far you have come or how close you are to achieving your goal. You will also need to find a way of congratulating yourself on celebrating your accomplishments after each routine check. This will serve to increase confidence in yourself.

Take a break to look at how much progress you have made.

Take a short break to look back on how much progress you have made so you can see the bigger picture. As you examine the data, pay attention to how consistently you've been able to fulfill your goals. Do you feel any different from how you felt before? These questions help you to determine what you have been doing right, and if there is anything you should be doing differently. This reflection creates room for you to analyze your newly formed routine of behavioral patterns so you can see if it is going to affect your lifestyle while allowing you to appreciate how far you have come in achieving your goals.

You might experience some obstacles that get in the way of you achieving your goal. One of the significant factors of CBT assignments and keeping a record of your progress is to allow you to recognize the obstacles that hinder you. This allows you to come up with effective strategies to tackle them. For instance, you might discover new ways of calming yourself during a panic attack by coming up with helpful thoughts that serve to soothe and stabilize you. Identifying these obstacles also helps you to come up with methods of ignoring and abandoning specific thought patterns that keep you from achieving your goals.

Goal setting and using a workbook

A goal-setting workbook is the perfect tool to help someone achieve his or her dreams and goals. It allows you to keep track of your progress and get things down on paper. A workbook allows you to:

· Keep a record of all your accomplishments

· Keep track of things you want to avoid doing

· Identify barriers keeping you from achieving your goal

· Keep a record of things that help get you through certain situations

· Set up long-term and short-term goals.

· Recognize areas needing improvements

· Come up with healthier routines

Chapter Four: Anxiety and Worry: CBT Techniques to Reduce Both NOW

Stress and worry are on the rise in our everyday life. Being always connected to the news, social media, and other aspects of the Internet has served to increase the risks of anxiety and worry. The increased pressure to achieve more, and uncertainty about our finances and career have also helped to contribute to increasing fear in people's lives. People now train themselves in the act of multitasking to do more work to meet daily needs, and this has only fostered anxiety. The mental health of the general population is at risk; now more than ever, the need to find a solution to the problems created by our society is on the increase.

Excessive worry, more often than not, leads to anxiety. Some people argue that worrying helps them to prepare for the unexpected, and while this may be true for certain people, for others it only leads to more problems.

Anxiety, worry, obsessive thoughts, and panic attacks are treatable. These mental health problems and other similar ones can all be managed to a level that allows you to lead a healthy life. Although medications for anxiety are quite useful to manage stress and worry, they only go as far as treating the symptoms. Anxiety therapy is the most effective course of treatment for anxiety, excessive fear, and panic attacks because, unlike medication, therapy goes as far as addressing the underlying cause of the mental health problem. It helps you discover the roots of your worries and fear while helping you come up with strategies on how to overcome them. It shows you how to look at the causes of your worries and anxiety in less frightening ways.

There different types of anxiety disorders, and each one is considerably different from another. This means that the particular therapy assigned for each one must be designed for the specific diagnosis and symptoms. The treatment plan for anxiety attacks will differ from those for a person with obsessive-compulsive disorder (OCD). The duration of time needed for therapy will also be dependent on the type and severity of anxiety disorder.

Many therapy techniques and types have been applied in treating anxiety disorder and excessive worrying, but the most effective approach is Cognitive Behavioral Therapy (CBT). Sometimes CBT is used together with other necessary therapy techniques depending on the need of the individual.

You must determine if your worry is either just the usual worry everyone has or excessive to the point of preventing you from leading a healthy life. Self-evaluation is essential to determine if your anxiety is a mental health problem. You can start by asking yourself the following questions.

Possibilities of Your Worries Coming True

What are the possibilities of what you are worried about happening?

You need to recognize what you are anxious and afraid of. For instance, if you are meant to give a speech, you might be concerned about people making fun and laughing at you. If you are worried about meeting with someone, it may be that you are afraid of what the person might say or that you may be rejected. If your worry is related to making mistakes at work, it might be that you are worried about being fired.

You have to be able to figure out what frightens you if you want to have any hope of overcoming anxiety. Most times, recognizing what you are terrified of will make you realize how baseless your fear is.

After determining the source of your fear, you need to determine the probability of your concern coming to pass. You need to logically analyze the times you have been in a similar situation and determine the number of times the worst-case scenario your fear predicts has come to pass. For instance, what is the likelihood of people making fun of you while you are giving a speech? Are there things you could do to decrease the probability of this happening? All these questions can make you realize that there are actual ways to influence the situation favorably.

Is the Best-Case Scenario Possible?

Sometimes people assume the worst-case scenarios when it comes to almost every situation. They have become experts in imagining the worst in everything, and as a result, they have forgotten that something contrary to their imagined scenario is possible. It is okay to consider the worst-case scenarios, and it might even prove to be useful, but when we forget about the best-case scenarios in every situation, then we might be taking our worries too far. You have to determine the two possible extremes of a scenario and then consider the most likely one. Most times, your mind wanders toward the more extreme scenarios while, in most cases, that doesn't happen. If you have difficulty determining the most likely scenario, it might do you good to imagine a situation with a mixture of both good and evil.

How Many Times Has Your Prediction Happened?

This is another useful way to determine if your actual worry is worthwhile by having a count of how many times the predicted worst-case scenario became a reality. If you are still okay, despite getting into a similar situation so many times over the years, this might mean your worry is baseless. Even if the worst-case scenario has happened before, you can compare the number of times it has happened to the number of times it hasn't. This can make you realize your fear might be unnecessary.

What Can You Do to Cope, even if the Worst Comes True?

Most times, you will see that your worry seems to go only towards the worst-case outcome. What comes after that seems not to be what worries us. It may be helpful to add "What happens next?" to your list of worries. This might help you figure out what you will do to cope if the worst-case scenario does happen. If you do get laughed at or made fun of when giving your speech, will you go home and sit in front of the TV all day or maybe sleep all day? Whatever the case might be, if you can extend your worry toward imagining a coping strategy, you will realize that you will be fine even after the worst-case scenario.

What Good Does Worrying About Every Situation Do?

This is the final question that you need to examine. Does worrying about the situation change the outcome? Does it make you any better at handling the outcome, or does it just make things worse? Sometimes worrying might serve to get you pumped up for the situation and prepare better. But too much worrying might do more harm than good. For instance, it might interfere with your preparations for an event; you might end up believing the worst-case scenario instead of looking at facts. No matter how much worry you put into the specific situation, the outcome cannot be influenced by it. So instead of worrying, you might as well spend your time doing things to prepare yourself better. Your worry might be self-defeating but focusing your mind and training your brain to address specific concern, you will become less likely to be taken over by your anxiety and worries.

This method of self-examination to determine if your worry and anxiety are doing you more harm than good is derived from Cognitive Behavioral Therapy. CBT has been proven to be the most effective method of therapy for obsessive worry and anxiety disorders.

Treating Obsessive Worry and Anxiety With CBT

CBT is based on the fact that our behaviors and feelings are dependent on our thoughts. People with anxiety disorders have a negative way of thinking that serves as a source of negative emotions, fear, and anxiety. CBT treatment of worry and anxiety helps you to recognize those negative thought patterns and correct them.

CBT for Anxiety - Thoughts to Challenge

This is referred to as cognitive restructuring. In this process, the negative thought pattern and beliefs of the individual with an anxiety disorder are challenged and replaced with more realistic and positive thoughts.

This process takes place in three steps.

Recognizing your negative thoughts

People with anxiety disorders often see the specific situation as being more dangerous than it actually is. For instance, individuals with germ phobia might be afraid of touching the handle of a door as it might be viewed as a threat to their lives.

Sometimes it is difficult to recognize or identify your irrational fear and thoughts. A way of achieving this is to ask yourself what your thoughts were when you were feeling anxious or worrying.

Challenging or addressing your negative thoughts

This is the second step, and it involves working with the therapist to come up with strategies for dealing with the thought triggers for your anxiety. To do this, you will have to come up with evidence of your negative thought pattern. You can obtain evidence by analyzing your distorted beliefs and putting your negative prediction to the test. The therapist will help you to come up with assignments that will allow you to do this and let you experiment with the advantages and disadvantages of various strategies as well as help you to realistically gauge the probability of your imagined worst-case scenario coming to pass.

Replacing negative beliefs and thoughts with positive, realistic ones

After the irrational fears and negative feelings that trigger your anxiety are identified, they can be replaced or modified to more positive and realistic ones. This is done with the help of your therapist, who will act as your guide to calm you when certain situations trigger your anxiety and panic attacks.

To give you a better understanding of thought-challenging with CBT, let's consider this example.

John is afraid of taking public transportation because he is afraid of dying in a commercial-vehicle disaster. After John's therapist recognized these negative thoughts, he asked John to write down his thoughts to identify the various distortions and errors in his thinking. Below is what he was able to come up with:

1. Persistent/Challenging Negative Thought:

What if I am in an accident and die while using a public transport system?

Cognitive distortion:

Predicting the worst-case scenario.

More Realistic thought:

The public transport system is used by a lot of my friends and family members who are still alive, so it must not be as unsafe as I think.

2. Second Negative Thought:

Dying in a transport accident is a terrible way of dying.

Cognitive distortion:

Not thinking straight.

More realistic thought:

There are a lot of ways to die; transportation accidents are just one of them; besides, even private transport can get involved in a road accident.

3. Third Negative Thought:

I could even die by just riding on any kind of public transport.

Cognitive distortion:

Jumping to conclusions.

More realistic thought:

People don't just die by getting on to public transport.

The process of replacing distorted negative thoughts with more positive and realistic ones is not an easy task. These distorted thoughts have been programmed into the mind of the individual in question and have become a pattern of thinking that can last a lifetime. It takes a lot of hard work to break any habit. CBT works hand in hand with the homework given to you to make it easier to achieve this. CBT for anxiety also include:

• Lessons to help you recognize when you become anxious by its effect on your body.

• Coping strategies to help you relax when dealing with anxiety and panic attacks.

• Challenging your fears (both imagined and real)

One system of homework or assignment that facilitates recovery from mental disorders and worries is known as Exposure therapy.

Exposure Therapy

A situation in which triggers anxiety is often unpleasant and people with anxiety disorders do whatever they can to avoid it as much as possible. For instance, if you are afraid of heights or plane flights, you will do whatever is within your power to avoid getting into any situation involving them. For those with the phobia of public speaking, they might even go as far as avoiding speaking at their best friend's wedding. In as much as these situations can be unpleasant, they can be an important aspect of living, and avoiding them takes away the chance for you to overcome them. And the more you avoid them, the stronger they become.

Exposure therapy aims to bring you into contact with those fearful situations and objects. It works on the theory that with repeated exposure, you will become accustomed to these situations and become more in control of your anxiety and panic attacks. There are two ways of achieving exposure therapy.

• Being asked by your therapist to imagine these scary objects and situations in sessions.

• Facing these situations in real life, so you can apply what you have gained in therapy sessions.

Systematic Desensitization

Sometimes facing your fears right away can lead to devastating results. Exposure therapy usually begins with situations that trigger mild anxieties and worries. It gradually works up from there toward more dangerous situations. This process of gradual exposure is known as systemic desensitization. It lets you build up tolerance and confidence for mastering control of your anxiety.

For instance, the process of systemic desensitization for fear of plane flights involves:

Step 1: staring at a picture of airplanes

Step 2: watching videos of aircraft in flight

Step 3: seeing a real plane taking off

Step 4: booking a flight ticket

Step 5: driving to the airport

Step 6: checking in for your flight

Step 7: getting on your plane

Step 8: taking the flight

Systematic Desensitization Occurs in Three-Phases

Learning relaxation skills

The first step involved in systemic desensitization is learning how to relax in those situations that trigger your anxiety. With the help of your therapist, you will be taught relaxing techniques like muscle relaxation and deep breathing. These techniques will be practiced both at home and in therapy sessions. These techniques will help reduce the physical symptoms (sweating, hyperventilating, and trembling) of your anxiety attacks as you confront your fears.

Create a step by step list

A list of those situations that trigger your anxiety will be created to help guide you toward your goal. A list of actions to overcome the fear of each situation will be made to provide a guide and strategy. Every step must be specific with a realistic and measurable objective.

Making anxiety therapy work for you

Anxiety needs a lot of hard thinking and time as well as commitment. Treatment with CBT requires you to face your fears, and sometimes you may end up feeling worse before getting better. But whatever the case may be, sticking to the treatment plan and listening to your therapist is paramount to your success.

Chapter Five: Dealing with Depression: CBT Tips to Feel Better Instantly

Life can get complicated at times, so it is perfectly normal to feel down once in a while. Feeling like everything is against you from time to time is an all too common feeling and one of the characteristics of being human, especially in today's society. According to a report by the Anxiety and Depression Association of America, 14.6 million people live with major depressive disorders.

Today many people work for longer hours only to receive the same pay; some have to deal with too many bills or personal relationship problems. Other people are dealing with addiction problems such as alcohol and drugs. Everyone has many issues, and not everyone is a hundred percent all the time. But when your feelings are at their lowest all the time to the extent that they impair your everyday life, or you experience feelings of despair that just won't go away; you might be experiencing depression. Depression is a dark and lonely place that can make day-to-day functioning a challenge. Some days you are overwhelmed, and the only solace you can find is in alcohol and drugs.

If you are in this place right now and feel like no one is coming to save you, the good news is you can help yourself. CBT had been proven to be extremely useful in helping people living with depression.

Types of Depression

Many people experience various kinds of depression. These different types of depression can be experienced either together or in addition to an addiction problem; whatever the case might be, CBT is useful for treating many kinds of depression.

Major Depression

This type of depression occurs when you have experienced five or more symptoms of depression for at least two weeks. Major depression is often weakening and interferes with a proper daily function such as work, sleep, eating, and studying. You can experience episodes of major depression a few times in your life. Sometimes they can happen as a result of traumatic events such as the death of a loved one or the breakdown of a relationship.

Bipolar Disorder

People with the type of depression experience symptoms of shifting moods. It involves a cycle which goes from feelings of mild to intense happiness (euphoria) to episodes of extremely overwhelming depression.

Persistent Depressive Disorder (PDD)

This type of depression was previously referred to as dysthymia. PDD is usually a less severe type of major depression, although its symptoms are often similar to that of major depression. People with this type of depression typically experience it for a least two years.

Some symptoms of PDD include stress, irritability, and the general lack of the ability to enjoy life.

Signs and Symptoms of Depression

Often, people are worried that they are experiencing depression. Because many people often feel sad from time to time, it is essential to be able to tell the difference between experiencing depression and just dealing with a short period of sadness. Depression can usually be identified by loss of interest in life in general and the inability to carry out daily functions effectively. The following signs and symptoms generally define depression.

- Lose interest in things you used to enjoy

- Constant feelings of helplessness and hopelessness

- Unexplainable tiredness

- Inability to concentrate, even when the task is easy

- Change in appetites — either eating more or less

- Failure to think anything positive.

- Aggressiveness, irritability, and short temper

- Drinking more alcohol than usual

- Engaging in reckless behavior

- Excessive use of prescribed or illegal drugs.

- Feelings of guilt and worthlessness, or self-loathing

Experiencing all of these symptoms is a sure sign of depression, and one of the best options of treatment available today for you is CBT.

Cognitive Behavioral Therapy for Depression

Having good knowledge of the symptoms and being able to identify them is the first step to recovery; many people sometimes find it difficult to identify signs of depression.

The next step is knowing about the various effective treatment plans for depression.

Cognitive-behavioral therapy is a psychotherapy that helps in modifying thought patterns to change negative moods and behaviors into more positive ones.

Treatment of depression with CBT applies both cognitive and behavioral therapy. With the help of your therapist, you will be able to identify those negative thought patterns that trigger inappropriate behavioral responses to certain situations.

The treatment plan follows a structured pattern to guide you in coming up with strategies to help you deal with those situations that serve as triggers. These strategies help in managing or eliminating your depression. CBT aims to improve your present state of mind rather than dealing with the past.

As with most mental illness, treatment of depression with CBT is a difficult task. To help you, below are some guidelines to help prepare you for treatment.

Therapy

Since CBT is a goal-oriented method of treatment, it doesn't require as much time as other methods of treatment. Therapy sessions could be once every week and could last for 30 or 60 minutes

The first set of therapy sessions will be used to determine if you need the treatment or are a fit for it and to know if you are comfortable with the procedure.

Although the main focus of CBT treatment is on your present life, your therapist will need some understanding of your past, so you will be asked some questions about your history and background.

You will make the final decision on the changes you want. Also, you and the therapist will make the decisions on what you want to be discussed each day.

CBT Treatment for Depression

With the help of your therapist, every one of your problems will be broken down into smaller, more manageable parts. Each part will be taken separately and solved following the laid-out plan. You will be asked to keep a record of your thoughts, emotions, feelings, and behavioral patterns to be able to identify and modify them.

The record will help your therapist determine how those thoughts, feelings, and emotions are affecting you, and to see which of them may be unrealistic and distorted. You will then work with your therapist to come up with strategies on how to cope with them, and then to gradually modify them.

You and your therapist will work together to come up with homework or assignments that will help you to practice and apply things learned in the sessions.

Further therapy sessions will provide the opportunity to see how much progress has been made so far from the previous session and to see how well the last assignment was accomplished.

Unlike other kinds of psychotherapy, CBT treatment requires a good relationship between the therapist and you, so every decision made will be made together. In order words during the procedure, no choice will be forced on you by the therapist.

Even after you are done with the sessions, you can continue to apply these strategies; this enables you to be healthy for as many years as possible.

How CBT Works for Depression

One of the unique features of CBT is that it requires less time, taking as little as 6 to 20 sessions.

During every session, you and your therapist will identify situations that contribute to depression and try to tackle those patterns of thought. The journal or diary used to keep records helps your therapist to break down those thought reactions and patterns into different groups such as:

All-or-nothing thinking, where your view of the world is black and white, or

Generalization of everything, which refers to using the result of an event to judge other events.

Automatic negative thought patterns, when certain circumstances trigger a series of negative thoughts which has become habitual.

Not believing the positive, when you always consider the prospect of any positive experience as something that can't possibly happen.

Minimizing or maximizing the importance of certain events, when the critical or non-critical natures of certain situations are distorted.

Blowing things out of proportion, wherein you always think everything that happens is as a result of what you have done or said, or that behaviors and activities of people are because of you.

Focusing on an adverse event, when you always tend to dwell on an adverse fact so that your view of reality is distorted

Keeping a record of things also helps you:

- To analyze yourself to come up with appropriate ways of responding to situations.
- To know how to talk to yourself in realistic ways.
- To be able to analyze your emotions and situations accurately.
- To be able to come up with appropriate responses to specific events.

Applying these methods and techniques help you to gain a balance with your mind and body.

How CBT Helps Depression

Depression has become one of the most widespread mental health problems experienced by both old and young, and the debilitating effects of depression can't be ignored. This mental health problem goes beyond affecting just your life; it also affects friends and family members. Depression is a common and severe illness that negatively impacts the lives of those close to the sufferer; family and friends as well as coworkers and employers.

Depression significantly affects the proper functioning of society as a whole. For example, when depression keeps you from carrying out your proper function at works and impacts your financial life, you won't suffer alone as the effects extend toward your family, employer, and anyone who tends to gain from you financially.

What Kinds of Depression does CBT Treat?

CBT is useful for treating people with moderate depression, and it can be used as a treatment plan without the need for medication. For those with significant depression, CBT works best when used together with drugs.

Just as depression affects both old and young, CBT is also effective in treating both, and it goes a long way toward reducing risks of relapse. The coping strategies and cognitive modifications derived from CBT treatment give you long term skills to deal with a lot of demanding situations. So, CBT is a useful tool to stay mentally healthy and free from depression for a long time.

For CBT to work, you must

· Be motivated to change your current situation

· Be capable of introspection

· Have the ability to control your reaction to things happening around you.

How the Components of CBT Work on Depression

CBT is a psychotherapy that has two components: the cognitive part and the behavioral part.

The cognitive part helps to identify those unrealistic negative thoughts that lead to negative behaviors and emotions. It also helps you to understand those beliefs that you have developed over time and what triggered their development. This is an essential part of CBT treatment for depression.

The behavioral part helps you to deal with treatment and modification of the various responses to and behavior in certain situations. With the help of your therapist, you will analyze your daily activities and their effects on your moods.

CBT goes beyond the therapy sessions as you will be given various assignments to practice everything gained in the therapy sessions.

Depression and Addiction

One of the most common associations of depression is an addiction. People who are depressed are at high risk for abuse and dependence on substances that numb those painful feelings. Sometimes abuse of specific substances such as alcohol depresses your central nervous system. Abuse of alcohol could, therefore, serve to induce depression. Twenty percent of Americans who suffer from anxiety and mood disorders like depression are addicted to alcohol or other substances.

Based on the statistics, it seems a fact that depression and addiction are closely related, and each of the condition tends to amplify the other. It is essential to seek help if you are experiencing both states at once.

The interrelationship between depression and addiction is referred to as dual diagnosis. People with both conditions often see life as being extraordinarily lonely and weakening, because both conditions serve to make the other worse.

Triggers of Depression and Addiction

Most times, it isn't easy to determine whether depression or addiction started first. But based on years of study and research, some triggers of both conditions have been identified.

Both conditions seem to affect the same area of the brain. This area of the brain is also responsible for how we respond to stress.

Genetic factors also have a significant role to play in substance abuse and depression. Certain people, due to their DNA, are more prone to depression and addiction.

Early development problems affect the mix; people who had mental health problems while growing up are more likely to become addicts, and people who had issues with substance abuse at an early age are more susceptible to mental health problems in the future.

Things to Remember About CBT

New experiences can be challenging, especially the life-changing ones, and going for CBT as your choice of treatment means you are going for something challenging. Doubts and worries about it working are perfectly normal, but you will be required to put in the work, and with the help of your therapist, a good result is guaranteed. Before going for CBT treatment for depression, it is essential to know the following.

· CBT explores those painful experiences and feelings that you always want to avoid, so you might end up facing these situations.

· Achieving your goal of having good mental health is totally up to you. Your therapist can only serve as a guide to encourage you, but in the end, you end up doing all the hard work.

· You will need to desire to be well, so you will have to push yourself even when you don't feel like it.

· If you want to get well, confronting those situations you normally try to avoid is going to be necessary.

Chapter Six: Workplace CBT: Ways to Beat Stress at Work

Concern for work-related stress is growing worldwide, and if you are worried about the amount of pressure you go through at work, then you are not alone. It is an issue that goes beyond just affecting the health of employees, impacting the efficiency and productivity of affected organizations. Many companies demand maximum commitment and have an enormous workload to be dealt with by their employees.

Many events serve as triggers for work-related stress. For instance, you might be overwhelmed with the workload you face, and the pressure of the demand it places on you to get it done might be impossible to deal with. Many jobs can require an absurd number of hours that you feel it isn't worth it. Different situations at work that can be a source of stress include:

· Work conflicts between colleagues or your employers

· Dealing with constant change at work

· Fear of losing your job or being demoted

Work pressure affects various individuals differently; not everyone has the same view of working. What you may view as challenging another person may see as extremely stressful while some other person might not feel it is much of either a challenge or stressful. This is because not everyone has the same psychological constitution. People have different experiences, and as a result don't always have the same views on certain things. But the fact remains that everyone feels stress when dealing with specific challenges in life.

Individual events can increase or decrease stress. Symptoms of work-related stress could be either physiological or psychological. Many individuals are searching for ways to reduce work-related stress. One method of dealing with stress that has proven useful in treating many aspects of psychological problems is cognitive-behavioral therapy (CBT). CBT helps people going through work-related stress to find a new perspective on their situation. It helps them manage pressure while also decreasing the effects of psychological and emotional stress. CBT also teaches new strategies to help them feel at ease and have more confidence in the face of any work challenge.

Identifying some specific symptoms of stress can be tricky, while other signs might be mild and manifest in smaller details. Whatever the case might be, you must recognize the symptoms of work-related stress to know when to seek help.

Symptoms of Work-Related Stress

Many studies have been carried out on the symptoms and effects of work-related stress

Symptoms such as upset stomach, headache, sleep problems, and relationship problems with friends and family are well-known signs of stress at work.

Symptoms of work-related stress are divided into three categories: psychological, physical, and behavioral.

Psychological Symptoms

· Depression

· Dermatological disorders

· Discouragement

· Pessimism

· Anxiety

· Irritability

· Cognitive difficulties

Some of these psychological problems are easy to identify. The physical effects of stress at work, on the other hand, are not so easy to recognize because they are associated with different problems and illness. Work-related stress may precipitate chronic disease. A study published by the Journal of Occupational and Environmental Mental Health revealed that the cost of health care is over 50 percent more for workers who experience high levels of work-related stress.

Cardiovascular Disease

Some jobs are extremely demanding and constantly changing, and do not give employees control over what is happening; these jobs increase the risk of cardiovascular disease.

Musculoskeletal disorders: specific jobs requiring certain forms of physical activity increase the risk for the development of diseases of the upper limbs and back.

Workplace injury: Stressful working conditions usually interfere with proper safety practices, increasing the risk of work-related injuries.

Suicide, cancer, ulcers, and immune function: According to some research, there exist some definite relationships between work-related stress and health problems such as these.

Physical Symptoms

- Headaches
- Fatigue
- Sleeping difficulties, such as insomnia
- Muscular tension
- Heart palpitations
- Gastrointestinal upsets, such as diarrhea or constipation
- High blood pressure
- Loss of appetite
- Poor job performance

Behavioral Symptoms

- Aggression
- An increase in sick days or absenteeism
- A drop in work performance
- Diminished creativity and initiative
- Mood swings and irritability
- Lower tolerance of frustration and impatience
- Disinterest
- Interpersonal relationships problems
- Isolation.
- Short attention span
- Procrastination
- Increased use of alcohol and drugs

Triggers of Work-Related Stress

These are some factors that act as facilitators for pressure at the workplace:

· Bad management

· High-performance demands

· Work environment and surrounding

· Lack of proper support

· Changes in management

· Trauma

· Role conflicts

Causes of Work-Related Stress

These factors are the major factors responsible for fear in the workplace.

· High workloads

· Long hours

· Short deadlines

· Job insecurity

· Changes within the organization

· Insufficient skills to get the job done

· Boring work

· Poor relationships with colleagues and employers

· Over-supervision

· Changes to duties

· Lack of proper resources

· Bad working environment

- Not enough promotion opportunities

- Lack of equipment

- Discrimination

- Harassment

- Random events in the workplace, such as workplace deaths.

How Does CBT for Stress Work?

CBT treatment for work-related stress helps in providing understanding about the effects of specific thinking patterns on our behavior and how those can raise your stress level. Also, while it helps you with identifying these thinking patterns, it helps you in creating new thinking patterns that change your behavior and response. It also serves to help boost your confidence and ability to cope with certain stressful and challenging situations

After going through cognitive behavioral therapy, you will be able to control your behaviors better and handle stressful situations with ease. You will also know how to prevent some situations at work being stressful at all.

Therapy

For the first CBT therapy session you will be asked various questions by your therapist, so the amount of help and the approach to take in handling the challenges you face can be determined. This also helps your therapist to come up with an appropriate plan to achieve the goal.

Subsequent sessions will be used to determine and identify the situations that act as triggers for you. This is done through a thoughtful discussion with your therapist. This helps you in knowing and seeing these triggers from a new angle. Also, you will learn new ways of thinking, handling, and coping with those stressful situations.

Various assignments will be given to you to help you put to work everything learned in the CBT sessions and to see how much your capacity for dealing with stressful situations at work has improved. There is no easy way out of work-related stress; you will have to put in a lot of hard work because these stressful situations are all stressful for a reason, and until you figure out how to deal with these reasons, your condition won't change.

Some practical tips from CBT which can help you in dealing with work-related stress include:

Learn to prioritize

Sometimes having too much on to do doesn't inspire you to do more; it may just add to an already stressful situation. You might end up feeling overwhelmed and feel like everything is out of your control.

You don't have to do everything. Learning how to prioritize is an essential aspect of working for some organizations — taking your time to prioritize makes things run more smoothly. You might even find out you have time for many other things that can serve to reduce work stress. You can make a list of the most important things to do as opposed to tasks that are not essential. This gives you a higher chance of being in control and taking your jobs one at a time from the most important to the least important.

Monitoring your mood

This is an essential tip of work stress management from CBT. Your therapist will help you in coming up with ways to control how certain situations and events at work affect your mood. In other words, it helps you to process how you feel towards particular circumstances while aiding you to see how some behavioral patterns affect your mood in specific ways.

When you find yourself focusing on particular thoughts like how much workload you face and worrying about yet-to-come situations at work, your mood-monitoring skill might come handy. You can get a journal to record your moods.

Record the stressful situation

Record how you feel at the time of the trigger situation or any time you think about the situation. You can rate each feeling based on how overwhelming it was.

Record everything you were thinking at the time of the situation. It is essential to get every single thought down, so you can tell how each one affects your feelings.

When you are done recording everything, you can put your journal away. After a few days, you can revisit your journal to go through what you had put down.

This way of recording everything that goes on with your thoughts and feelings is a great way to teach yourself to see your emotions from another angle. You are more likely to notice just how distorted your views and attitudes were at the time of the situation when you visit your journal a few days later. This gives you the chance to be better able to recognize which thoughts need modifying and changing so next time you can better deal with and respond to the situation.

From CBT, you can learn how these negative thought patterns (cognitive distortions) affect your mental health and how we can come up with strategies for dealing with them.

Focus on the things you can control and develop a positive balance

In situations where we feel overwhelmed and consumed by our workload, we often tend to focus only on things we can control. This often ends up raising our overall stress level and exhausting our minds, using up energy that we could be using to achieve something better.

In times like this, CBT lessons for reframing our minds and thinking can help us feel in control.

Positive reframing is different from just positive thinking. Positive reframing helps you come up with new ways and strategies using the facts available to look at things in a more realistic manner. Instead of just coming up with positive thinking towards the stressful situation or task, positive reframing comes up with an alternative way of solving or coping with the situation. For instance, you could be in charge of planning the end-of-year party for your organization/company and, at the same time, managing your already busy schedule. Positive reframing could help you come up with an alternative way by helping you see the importance of delegating instead of just handling everything yourself

Situation: a big upcoming event that requires a lot of details and inputs. Thoughts: *This is so much work for me; I don't think this work can be just for me. Doing this alone could result in a big disaster.*

Emotions: irritable, depressed, and anxious.

Behaviors: avoid everything to do with it. Avoid doing the project, procrastinate, and leave out important details of the project.

Alternative thought: *Although this is a lot of work for one person, I have always been good at accomplishing jobs like this, and for me to be assigned this task means my boss thinks highly of me, which means I can do this and must not disappoint. I'm going to do every bit of research required for this task; this could be my chance to show my stuff. I can always ask for help if I'm stuck, so I will carry it out diligently to see how far I can go on my one for now.*

Look for satisfaction and meaning in your work

Sometimes we may end up feeling dissatisfied and bored with the constant stream of work. This is a significant cause and source of stress for many people and can affect your mental and physical health. Some of us have always dreamed of the perfect position, career, or job. One of the greatest motivations and source of drive that get many people going is being passionate about their work. Once this is lost, you are going to feel dissatisfied.

Maybe you are not in your dream job, but you can still find purpose in being there. With ambition, you can even learn to develop a passion for the job. Even in some extremely unimportant tasks, you can learn to find meaning in the little contributions you make. All you have to do is focus your attention on the aspects of the job you love and enjoy. Even if it doesn't seem like much to others, you might find out that with time you might get the promotion you seek.

At other times, when you feel helpless and uncertain, when the level of your stress is over the roof, some of the tips below can be of help to you:

Speak to your employer about workplace stressors

Your employers are aware that happy employees of sound mind are more efficient and productive, so they will always try their best to tackle work stress to get the best out of the employees. So, it is important to let your employers know of those stressors that makes it impossible to carry out your job effectively

Get a clear description of your job

If you don't have a good understanding of your responsibilities and duties concerning a task, you might find the task very difficult. This can increase the level of your work-related stress. You can always ask for clarification on a mission, so you know what you are doing.

· You can ask for a transfer into another department to escape the toxic environment.

· If you are tired, bored, or stressed out by the same old task, you can ask for something new.

Chapter Seven: Intrusive Thoughts: Acknowledging and Eliminating Them with CBT

Sometimes you might experience specific thoughts that pop into your head from nowhere. Maybe you're just going about one of your daily activities, and suddenly your mind comes up with a bizarre thought or crazy image, leaving you wondering where it came from. Most of the time, the idea could be harmless such as doing something stupid and socially crazy in public. Sometimes it could be a thought that could do more harm than good, or something that you could never dream of doing, like pushing someone down a flight of stairs.

The good news is you are not the only one experiencing strange and bizarre thoughts popping into the mind at random times.

What are Intrusive Thoughts?

Intrusive thoughts are thoughts that come into our consciousness without any prompting or warning. The contents of these thoughts are sometimes usually unacceptable to the general population, as they are disturbing and alarming or just weird. When these thought gets stuck in our head for some reason, they can lead to severe distress.

In some situations, where such thoughts occur frequently, they may start interfering with our everyday life. These thoughts could be of behaviors that are violent in nature, sexual, and other disturbing fantasies that are unacceptable to you.

It is essential to know these thoughts are nothing more than thoughts and have no meaning whatsoever, so the power they have over you will be only that which you give to them. When you focus more attention than is necessary on these thoughts and get worried over them, feeling ashamed and becoming disturbed by them, then you could be experiencing a mental disorder.

When you know that these thoughts are nothing but thoughts, and you have no obligation to do as they suggest, intrusive thoughts can't be harmful.

What Causes Intrusive Thoughts and Are They Normal?

The cause of intrusive thoughts hasn't been determined for sure, but some psychologists have published some theories. Lynn Somerstien proposed that maybe the reason for these thoughts surfacing is because the person is going through something difficult. This situation could be interpersonal problems, work stress, parent and parenting problems, or something which the person is trying to keep under wraps. Unfortunately, instead of the thoughts of these problems staying buried, they find an alternative way of manifesting.

Another psychologist who has proposed another theory is Dr. Hannah Reese. She suggested that the manifestations of these thoughts are a result of our failure to act in the way they suggest, because while you will never do as these thoughts suggest, your brain goes right on coming up with some of the most bizarre things it can imagine.

This brings us to the question of why our brain keeps coming up with such thoughts.

Dr. Sally Winston and Dr. Martin Seif came up with an outstanding description of what they believe causes intrusive thoughts. They believe that our brains create what they call "junk thoughts" and these are part of the debris that floats around in our stream of consciousness. Thoughts like these are meaningless, and if we avoid them and ignore them, they just disappear.

The argument of where these intrusive thoughts come from remains a mystery, but the fact remains that in some cases people dwell too much on them, and the more they try to avoid it, the more they think about it.

In some other cases, these thoughts come as a result of an underlying mental health problem or a brain problem such as

· Post-traumatic stress disorder (PTSD)

· Obsessive-Compulsive Disorder (OCD)

· Brain injury

· Parkinson's disease

· Dementia

It is essential to notice changes or symptoms in your mental health because they are not to be taken lightly. Some early signs of mental health problems include

· Changes in thought patterns

· Thoughts of disturbing imagery

· Obsessive thoughts

For instance, if someone tells you to avoid thinking of a green whale, even though you are allowed to think about anything else in the world, don't think about a green whale, it can be hard avoiding the thought of a green whale, especially for a long time. In time you will find that your mind will slip up and the image of a green whale will come to mind.

In a healthy mental state, it is easy for you to monitor and keep track of your many thoughts, and even when the little random reflections come up, it is easy to let them slip away.

In situations where you find it difficult to let go of these intrusive thoughts but instead you keep on focusing on them more and more frequently; then it is essential to seek help.

Intrusive Thoughts and Other Mental Health Disorders

Some of the mental disorders most associated with intrusive thoughts include:

· Anxiety;

· OCD;

· Depression;

· TSD;

· Bipolar Disorder;

· ADHD

Intrusive thoughts popping up in our minds is normal; everyone experiences it. However, in cases where they come up more frequently and lead to significant distress you may have one of the associated mental disorders mentioned above.

Intrusive Thoughts and OCD

One of the significant easily recognized symptoms of OCD is frequent intrusive thoughts, experienced by almost all persons diagnosed with OCD.

According to Dr. Robert L. Leahy, these thoughts are often evaluated negatively: You might end up thinking that there is something wrong with you because these thoughts which you should not be thinking of keep popping into your mind. So, the only way you see of controlling them is to pay close attention to them, to monitor and prevent them from coming up.

People with OCD who experience these compulsive intrusive thoughts react in a certain way to these thoughts, leading to more severe problems. The frequency of these thoughts only escalates with more attention paid to it, leading to them becoming an obsession. This obsession results in repeated behaviors carried out in order to avoid the recurrence of these thoughts.

Some examples of intrusive thoughts relating to OCD include worrying about shutting the windows, having the key to the door, and worrying about batteries on surfaces. Someone with OCD may develop the habit of cleaning surfaces multiple times or avoid touching the handle of the door or rechecking repeatedly to be sure they have their keys with them. These compulsions often affect the quality of life of the individual and interfere with a healthy daily life.

Intrusive Thoughts and Depression

People suffering from depression are also prone to having intrusive thoughts. Frequent depressive intrusive thoughts can also cause depression. When too much attention is placed on specific negative and depressive intrusive thoughts that frequently occur (rumination), it can lead to severe depression. You might return time and time again trying to address these thoughts, but instead of solving the issue you only end up making it worse.

Some examples of intrusive thought within depression include:

· Placing too much focus on negatives and always expecting worst-case scenarios.

· Placing too much emphasis on a specific horrible event and using it as a reference to other similar events in the future.

· Over-analyzing things in your head (over-thinking)

· Always assuming you know what others are thinking

· Accepting the worst-case scenario as the only possible outcome of a particular situation

· Exaggeration of a certain event

· Taking responsibility for things that you can't control

Thoughts like these can cloud your mind and make it impossible for you to see things as they actually are. Instead of seeing most of what goes on in your head as just thoughts, you end up believing them, taking every analysis as real and not being objective in your conclusions.

Intrusive Thoughts and Anxiety

In cases of OCD, the person involved tends to experience intense graphic, violent, and unacceptable intrusive thoughts, while people with anxiety often feel like they are drowning in many unwanted thoughts of less intensity than those of OCD sufferers.

In the case of a Generalized Anxiety Disorder (GAD), patients may experience uncontrollable worry about the safety of a loved one. Certain people with an anxiety disorder relating to fear of social situations (social phobia) might find it challenging to get over memories of making a mistake or saying something they shouldn't have said.

Usually when someone with an anxiety disorder experiences an intrusive thought, they will end up making the worst decision concerning the negative feeling. They often spend more time than is necessary obsessing over the thought, all in the name of trying to get it out of their mind. When they spend additional time on an intrusive thought, they often give it power over them, losing control over their minds as a result.

Intrusive Thoughts and PTSD

Another mental health problem strictly associated with intrusive thoughts is post-traumatic stress disorder (PTSD). In the case of PTSD, the intrusive thoughts are related to a particularly traumatic event that has already taken place, and could even involve flashbacks to it.

People with PTSD have difficulty forgetting what has happened in the past to them; as a result, the symptoms of PTSD make them deal with the past over and over again. They experience flashbacks from time to time in the form of nightmares and intrusive thoughts. In episodes of PTSD, the state of the body is similar to that of the previous situation. As a result, the person is on high alert due to floods of the "fight and flight" hormones and other hormones to the brain.

Intrusive Thoughts and ADHD

A primary symptom of ADHD is intrusive thoughts. People with ADHD often find it difficult to pay attention, even in the most conducive of environments. Difficulty concentrating is a general feature of this mental health condition, and one cause for this is frequent disturbing intrusive thoughts. People with ADHD experience a higher degree of intrusive thoughts than those with OCD even though the disorders are similar.

Cognitive Behavioral Therapy (CBT) Treatment for Intrusive Thoughts

CBT is one of the most effective treatment options for intrusive thoughts. Since intrusive thought has to do with how these how random thoughts pop into the mind and influence behavior, CBT is nothing short of a perfect choice of treatment for this mental health condition. CBT is used alone or in combination with other options of treatment depending on the severity of the condition.

CBT helps in creating and coming up with management strategies for dealing with harmful and undesired thoughts and behaviors. Through CBT, you will be able to learn how to come up with healthier ways of ignoring intrusive thoughts.

Acceptance and Commitment Therapy (ACT)

Acceptance and Commitment Therapy is a subtype of CBT that teaches you to accept your feelings and thoughts instead of engaging in a battle to avoid them. ACT shows you how to be mindful while coming up with alternative ways of thinking. It teaches people with these intrusive thoughts to accept these thoughts as normal but not to dwell on them as they are just one of many thoughts that can be ignored. The six principles of ACT are:

Cognitive Diffusion: You learn to give little weight to negative thoughts, emotions, and images.

Acceptance: learning how to let those intrusive thoughts run through your mind without feeling distressed

Contact the present moment: learning to focus on the current instead of overthinking the past or the future, and learning to accept things going on around you.

Observing yourself: Being aware or conscious of your being.

Values: identifying those important values your life is based on, those things you find the most important.

Committed action: Assigning goals depending on your values and the things you are fighting for.

These six principles help in treating and healing you while creating a forward-thinking mind.

Exposure and Response Prevention (ERP)

Another aspect of CBT that has proven effective in helping people with OCD achieve stable mental health is Exposure and Response

Prevention (ERP). In this method of therapy, you are exposed to the situations and events that act as triggers of your fear, and learn how to deal with them better.

ERP aims to show you that you are capable of challenging those fears, so you will come to realize how irrational they are. Those intrusive thoughts might remain, but with the help of this therapy, they become nothing more than a negligible nuisance that you don't pay much mind.

Self-Help: Managing Intrusive Thoughts with CBT

This method is used in addition to other CBT methods to lessen the symptoms of intrusive thoughts and give you a better quality of life when faced with intrusive thoughts.

According to Seif and Winston (2018), there are seven steps that can help you in changing your attitude towards intrusive thoughts and in getting over them.

- Give these thoughts a label, such as "intrusive thoughts".

- Know that you don't have control over these thoughts, they are automatic.

- Do not push the thoughts away, accept them.

- Float, and pass away the time.

- There is no need for a rush. Give yourself time, remember that less is more.

- The thoughts will come again, expect them.

- You can allow the anxiety to be present, but do not stop what you were doing before the intrusive thought.

Also, Seif and Winston put up some warning signs against these thoughts.

- Engage the thoughts in the best way you can.

- Do not keep the thoughts in your mind.

- Find the meaning of the thought.

- Observe to see if this is effective in getting rid of the thoughts.

The North Point Recovery center, which is an organization that helps people dealing with various disorders and substance abuse, came up with five tips to help people in challenging their intrusive thoughts.

- Take a more in-depth view of why intrusive thoughts bother you.

- Don't block your mind. Allow the thoughts in and move on from them.

- Don't be triggered by thoughts; they are just thoughts, don't give them more power than they have.

- Don't react emotionally to intrusive thoughts.

- Trying to align your behaviors with your obsession won't help in the long run.

Chapter Eight: Mindfulness and the CBT Connection

With the increase in popularity of both CBT and MCBT treatments for various mental health issues, many questions have been asked about what the two offer the world of psychology. The more popular Cognitive Behavioral Therapy (CBT) has gained a broad audience for its practical and goal-oriented method of dealing with many illnesses. The relative newcomer, MBCT, still has a long way to go to attain the popularity of CBT.

Because of the many values and similarities, it is often difficult to tell the difference between the two methods.

To give you a full picture of the basic principles and what both methods of psychotherapy are about, we are going to go through a summary of both approaches.

Cognitive-Behavioral Therapy (CBT)

For this comparison, we are going to go through a short overview of CBT, which we've already seen in chapter one.

As the name implies, Cognitive Behavioral Therapy is a type of psychotherapy that applies two components of treatment: the

Cognitive and the Behavioral components. By using these two parts in its goal-oriented treatment plans, it has been successful in treating various mental health problems such as anxiety disorders, PTSD, depression, schizophrenia, and OCD, among others.

Cognitive component: the cognitive component is the part of CBT responsible for recognizing those distorted thoughts and modifying them into more realistic ones. You might be experiencing specific thoughts and feelings that serve to make you have some distorted beliefs. When you act on this unrealistic belief it often leads to specific behaviors that can interfere with healthy living and many aspects of life, such as the relationship between family members, romantic relationships, academics, and work.

For instance, when someone suffers from low self-esteem, they might be dealing with some distorted (negative) thoughts about their capabilities and appearance. This could result in negative thinking patterns that might tend to keep them away from social events or give up specific opportunities that involve dealing with or exposure to people.

The cognitive component of CBT addresses the actions of modifying and changing these destructive thoughts. With the help of your therapist, you will be able to identify those distorted thought patterns and beliefs. This stage of CBT is referred to as "functional analysis". This stage is vital, so you can move forward with determining how these thoughts affect your behavior.

Behavioral Component

This part of CBT deals with the resulting behaviors due to the distorted negative thoughts. These behaviors are the end products of false and unrealistic beliefs due to negative thinking patterns. With the help of the behavioral component, you will be shown a new skill or strategy for coping with these behaviors, which can be applied to actual life situations.

In most cases, a change of behavior is accomplished in many gradual steps.

An instance of CBT in action would be when you are supposed to go out with a friend and he turns you down, saying he is busy. You might end up thinking that he hates you and so wants to stay away from you, especially if this happens repeatedly. This leads to more negative thinking, leading to you doubt and question your worth. You might end up feeling anxious and paranoid, so the next time you have an outing you end up using your previous experience to judge it.

In CBT treatment, you will be taught how to recognize and identify these negative thoughts. Instead of believing them, you will be shown how to look at an alternative pattern of analyzing the situation. You will learn how to question all your negative assumptions. You will be asked to consider the other previous outing you have had with your friends or someone. After going through all these, maybe you will be shown that perhaps all these thoughts are just in your head, and perhaps the friend who turned you down is indeed just busy.

What is Mindfulness?

It is a widespread belief that our reality is defined by the way we think. It's also believed that this reality can be influenced by improving the quality of one's thoughts. Every thought and feeling you experience shapes the nature of your reality. Mindfulness-based cognitive therapy, or MBCT, helps you recognize and understand the tone of your thoughts and feelings and to create new, healthy habits.

MBCT effectively combines cognitive therapy along with techniques of mindfulness to help an individual deal with issues like anxiety, depression, or any other behavioral problems. It mainly helps lessen your worries, stress, and fears by enabling you to control your emotions.

The ability to be aware of the thoughts popping into your head without getting carried away by them is known as mindfulness. The mind tends to wander, and as you try to concentrate on the task at hand, you might notice other thoughts creeping in. Mindfulness enables you to control your mind by using techniques that encourage you to take stock of your thoughts and decide whether you want to respond to them or not.

Mindfulness psychotherapy is designed to make you focus your awareness on the present moment. It helps you to analyze your feelings, thoughts, and bodily sensations calmly.

The foundation of mindfulness is based on an ancient technique used by Buddhist and specific Eastern spiritual teachings, and is designed to help people in attaining awareness of their body, feelings, and mind in order for them to gain self-actualization.

Mindfulness was developed in the 1970s by Dr. Jon Kabat-Zinn, who was the head of a stress reduction clinic at the University of Massachusetts. It was used as a psychological tool in the control of stress, anxiety, and chronic pain. It was researched and used in the treatment of depression in the 1990s. Today MBCT has been scientifically researched and is recognized by many of the world's leading psychologists, doctors, and scientists.

Mindfulness has been useful in helping people in dealing with the "auto-pilot" life we live in today's modern world. It helps us in always staying conscious of the present. This is important when dealing with mental illness like depression. Allowing the subconscious to rule over our lives gives room for a specific psychological condition like anxiety to come into our life. Getting distracted can leave us open to being taken over by particular challenges. If this happens, our reaction to it is bound to be automatic, and we can overreact and go off the rails. When we are ever-conscious of our present and aware of everything around us, we have a higher chance of responding calmly to individual challenges, events, or situations.

With the help of mindfulness, we think carefully, considering every option available before responding or acting. So, before acting, we consciously acknowledge the people, environment, and everything that will be affected by our action.

What is MBCT?

Mindfulness-Based Cognitive Therapy (MBCT) is a combination of various aspects of Cognitive Behavioral Therapy and mindfulness.

According to the two psychologists, Philip Barnard and Jon Teasdale, the human mind is made of two different modes, the "*being*" mode and "*doing*" mode. They described the "doing" mode as goal-oriented, and it is active when you come across a difference between how you want a thing to be and how the situation presents. The "being" mode, on the other hand, accepts situations the way they are without doing anything to change them. They further went on to say that the "being mode" is the one associated with long-lasting emotional changes. So, it was concluded that for cognitive therapy to be effective it will have to support not only cognitive awareness like CBT, but also the "being mode" of the mind. They believed that cognitive therapy could only be effective when used in combination with mindfulness.

A combined effort of psychiatrists Jon Kabat-Zinn, Zindel Segal, and Mark William helped in combining the various new ideas of cognitive therapy with the mindfulness-based stress reduction program of Kabat-Zinn. This led to the birth of MBCT.

The goal of MBCT is similar to that of CBT in that it helps you in maintaining a constant awareness of your reactions and thoughts. This enables you to notice any change that occurs due to negativity. But MBCT includes something extra in that it shows you how to become aware of time or moments when you are triggered by any negativity.

With this, you can better manage and control anxiety and stress by becoming more aware of what is happening at the present moment.

So instead of putting so much attention on trying to understand your thoughts, with MBCT you accept it for what it is without any judgment; you just let it go through your mind without paying much attention or attaching much meaning to it.

More awareness of the present moment means it is less likely you will be caught off guard by any trigger, so you can easily detach yourself from worries or moods.

Difference between CBT and MBCT

With the help of CBT, you can identify and modify patterns of negative thoughts that often cause anxiety and depression.

On the other hand, MBCT teaches you how to identify negative thoughts and to know for a fact that these thoughts are only thoughts, and nothing more. MBCT also goes further in applying mindfulness to be aware of what is happening in the present moment, such as your current thought, your present feelings, and everything you are experiencing in the present. It helps you not to be caught off guard by any negative thinking.

CBT applies cognition to understand how negative thought works. It is often described as "a thinking therapy"; it analyzes your thoughts, emotions, and reactions. Although it takes account of the response of your body to the stress of negative thoughts, it is a therapy that deals mainly with the thinking process. The main focus of CBT is on you mentally avoiding negative thoughts.

The techniques applied in MBCT are a little different from those used in CBT; they involve things like focus on breathing, where a few minutes is spent with your attention solely on the process of your breath, and body scans, where time is spent observing the different sensations and tensions in your body during sitting meditations. Because of these techniques, it is often referred to as "a feeling process". MCBT is, therefore, both experimental and analytical; it is more focused on the body than CBT. The pivotal point of MBCT is allowing your thoughts to come and then letting them go.

Similarities between CBT and MBCT

· Some similarities between CBT and MBCT include:

· Both methods help you to manage your thoughts properly.

· They both make you more resistant to automatic thought patterns, reactions, and feelings.

· Both methods of treatment require only a short time to achieve their goals.

· They are both best suited as the only method of treatment for mild anxiety and depression, unlike treatment plans for abuse and trauma that might require more than one form of therapy and a longer time of treatment

It is important to note that both methods of treatment are more beneficial after a successful application of talk-therapy treatment. MBCT is the more helpful of the two for people who have long-term depression and need a remedy for recent episodes of depression. Even after the therapy is over, negative thoughts are still connected to negative moods in your brain and could be triggered again. So being able to monitor those triggers and your views around situations that serve as triggers is a technique MBCT provides.

Benefits of MBCT

More control over your thoughts

MBCT has helped a lot of people with various mental health issues. Currently, it is applied to teach people how they can better understand their thoughts, patterns, and mechanisms. This helps them to recognize the signs and symptoms that point towards a mental health issue.

MBCT encourages you to be mindful of the present in general, not only during the time of therapy sessions and while doing meditations. This enables you to live outside your head, to pay more attention, and connect with people around you. With this way of living, you are less likely to encounter any negative thoughts that might lead to a mental health problem. People who practice MBCT let go of any depressive thoughts instead of holding on to them.

Stress reduction

In addition to meditation, deep breathing is another practice of mindfulness that is embedded in MBCT. A deep breath is a useful technique that calms the nervous system in times of stress. This can come in handy in times when you have the urge to react to those stressors.

Stress, in general, can be reduced with the help of MBCT because it gives the ability to become more aware of yourself in the present. So, your attention is focused on the matters at hand, giving no free time to excessive thinking and worrying about certain situations in the future or past. These factors have enabled MBCT practitioners to be more resistant to stress and to deal better with any stressful situation.

Improved mood

With the joint effort of both CBT and MBCT, you can learn to improve your mood and deal with depression. Even people with anxiety and depression can learn how to apply techniques from MBCT to prevent those minor feelings of sadness from turning into a deeper state of grief.

Constant practice of mindfulness has proven to be useful in helping people connect to their purpose in life; thus, they have no time to feel worthless or lost. This is because mindfulness teaches people to be and live in the present and be more thankful for everyday life . When you pay more attention to what is going on presently rather than letting yourself be carried away with thoughts or worries and external distractions, you will not only be more thankful; you will also notice your value to the world. Some studies have shown mindfulness to be useful in developing the area of the brain that reduces anxiety and increases positive feelings

CBT and MBCT have been proven through many studies and much research to be exceptional in treating depression and anxiety, among many other mental health issues. If you are confused about which therapy method would be suited to you, ask the opinion of your therapist.

Chapter Nine: Three Mindfulness Meditation Techniques You Should Know

Mindfulness makes it easy to understand your thoughts as well as behavioral patterns. It encourages you to appreciate the little joys of life without getting bogged down by the usual stress. By being mindful, you will be more adjusted and less judgmental towards yourself, others, and any situations in life. By figuring out the connection between the downward spiral and negative thinking, you will no longer feel helpless and will be better equipped to deal with your life. It encourages you to stop harboring ridiculously high expectations from yourself while enabling you to love yourself for who you are.

From the previous chapter on mindfulness and its connection with CBT, you should have understood how mindfulness meditation is an effective way to manage our feelings of stress and anxiety. It can be used to achieve a relaxed state during panic attacks, as mindfulness helps to slow down racing thoughts while focusing on the present, letting go of negativity, and calming both your mind and body. For a better understanding of these techniques, let's start with understanding meditation itself.

Basics of Meditation

Meditation entails staying in a relaxed position and concentrating your psyche on one idea while clearing it of all others. Your concentration might be on a sound, or your breathing, counting, or on nothing at all. A desirable aspect of meditation is that the mind does not follow every new thought that comes to the surface. Meditation, being popular, definitely has different forms and styles but all still follow specific patterns as explained below:

Keeping a quiet mind

A lot is going on in our world, and it is quite hard to keep our thinking mind quiet. However, with meditation, it is possible to keep the voices down. This means you are not focused on the things in your daily dealings that put you in a state of stress, not concentrating on your life's problems. You should know that without constant practice, you will find it hard to turn off these voices inside your head.

Being in the moment

It is essential that you learn how to keep your mind focused on the present. This is possible with meditation as all forms of meditation involve focusing on the present. You being in the present consists of experiencing each moment, then letting it go, and then moving onto the next. This takes a whole lot of practice, as focusing on the moment can be difficult because of the amount of time we spend thinking about the future or contemplating the past.

It is worth noting that meditation is widely advertised as a health-boosting practice. The reasons for this are mentioned below:

Health benefits

Meditation has provided a whole lot of positive benefits, from reducing stress symptoms to enhancing immunity. It reduces episodes of depression and anxiety. It also improves concentration.

Social Benefits

It has been reported to help improve relationships and also to enhance creativity. This goes a long way to reduce cases of low self-esteem and self-judgment, which reduce individual productivity. Having these benefits helps you to give your best in whatever situation comes your way, be it at work, school, or at home.

Cost-effective

Meditation is not one of those self-care practices that require a lot of funding; it is practically free. Your income cannot keep you from enjoying all the benefits to be had from meditation.

Productivity

Meditation only requires a few minutes (as few as five minutes!) daily to produce all its benefits.

Putting all these reasons together, it becomes easier for you to see why meditation has become a popular complement to medical practices today.

Mindfulness Meditation

Mindfulness involves focusing on the present moment rather than thinking about the future or the past. It could be focusing on a particular sensation, not for the sake of you examining the sensation but to experience it as it is. Another example is focusing on an object, not to place judgment on it but to savor the experience of the sensation you are getting from it. In other cases, you could focus on your breathing.

Certain individual components are crucial to practicing mindfulness meditation. These components include:

Focus

This is your ability to selectively place your attention or awareness on just one of the many sensations currently bombarding your mind or body, for an extended period without getting distracted. Imagine the thousands of feelings that are coming to you right now; the wind blowing against your skin, the sound of the overhead fan, the humming of the air conditioner, the pressure from the surface you are sitting on, the taste of your mouth, the rising and falling of your belly, etc. All these are demanding your attention, and it is an outstanding skill to be able to focus on just one for some time without getting distracted. This is usually hard for most people as the world we live in is overflowing with lots of things to catch our attention as we go through our activities at work and home. It has become a hard thing to sit down to read a book for just 10 minutes!

This is going to take a lot of practice but will be worth it. It is advised that you stay away from distractions like the computer, TV, radio, and your smartphone when performing mindfulness meditation.

Sensory Clarity

The next component speaks to how well you understand the information being passed from the raw data being assembled by your mind. Sometimes, what we think we know of particular situations is not so, and these misconceptions can lead to unnecessary anxiety. So, it is crucial that you calmly understand your situation before you act. This may be likened to looking through a microscope; at first, you see through lower magnifications. Later on, after a thorough understanding of the specimen at that magnification, you can change the lens to one of higher magnifications for better appreciation of the sample. This is to tell you that the more you practice, the clearer you see.

Equanimity

This is a critical ability that involves experiencing emotions and sensations without being affected by or reacting emotionally to them. This ability is a form of "decentering", which is paying attention to and accepting all thoughts coming in, but nevertheless not reacting to them.

Mindfulness Meditation Techniques

These techniques all follow specific procedures; taking notice of a particular sensation, labeling its channel of awareness, and savoring its experience without placing judgments. "Channel of awareness" is in regard to how you have become aware of the feeling being focused on. At this point, you need to understand the distinction between inner and outer awareness. These channels are seen in both inner and outer awareness, and they include:

Seeing

Outer seeing speaks to images of objects formed on the retina of the eyes while internal seeing is in regard to your imagination.

Hearing

Outer hearing occurs through our ears, while the inner awareness is playing a tune in our mind or engaged in internal monologue.

Feeling

The external feeling talks of the various stimuli you can sense within and without your body, while the inner feeling talks of your emotions such as nervousness, fear, anger, sadness, happiness, joy, etc.

That said, some analytical techniques that you should know include:

Three-Minute Breathing Space

To perform this exercise, you can either stand, sit, or lie down. Find a comfortable position to get started with this exercise. The first step is to become fully aware of yourself. Concentrate on what is going on in your mind and how you are feeling. Stop whatever activity you were engaged in and shift all your awareness back to your body, thoughts, feelings, and your breathing. Avoid moving your body and slowly concentrate on yourself.

While doing this, you might come across specific negative thoughts or beliefs present in your mind. Whenever you come across any negativity, don't try to ignore or avoid it. Instead, allow yourself to feel whatever you are feeling. Don't try to change anything at this stage. Instead, acknowledge these thoughts and allow them to pass. Now, repeat this step for any other feelings or sensations present in your body. Whenever you notice tension in a specific part of your body, acknowledge it and move on.

The second part of this exercise is to concentrate on one thing, and that is the way you breathe. Breathe in and focus on the way your abdomen moves. Whenever you inhale, your abdomen pushes upward, and when you exhale, it falls. Allow this step to anchor your thoughts and let the grounding effect wash over you. Once you have managed to gather and concentrate your thoughts and energy on yourself, you can start focusing the sense of awareness along the length of your body.

To perform this exercise, you can set a timer if you want. By setting a timer for three minutes, you will know when to start and end the exercise. The great thing about this exercise is that it can be performed anywhere at any time. Whenever you start feeling anxious, stressed, or even worried, take a break from whatever activity you are engaged in and concentrate on your breathing.

Mindfulness stretching

A great thing about the practice of mindfulness is that you can do this all day long, and it can easily be incorporated into your exercise routines as well. Before you start exercising, always concentrate on stretching your body. It helps relieve any tension or anxiety present within. Stretching is crucial because it helps reduce the risk of any injury while improving your physical performance. Apart from this, it also helps re-energize your body and prepare it for the exercise that lies ahead. Whenever you stretch, there is an increase in the supply of blood as well as oxygen to all the cells in your body.

Mindfulness stretching also increases your state of awareness while bringing about balance to your physical body.

Pandiculation might sound like a complicated process, but it is a simple stretching exercise. There are three simple stages in this exercise. The first step is to pay attention to the muscles in your body while voluntarily contracting them. The second phase is to release these muscles slowly, and the third stage is relaxation. You can perform this exercise wherever you are, even when you are lying down. Try to contract all the muscles in your body, slowly release them, and then feel relaxation wash over you.

While stretching, ensure that you are stretching the right muscles; avoid placing unnecessary stress on your joints or muscles, and stretch slowly. By following these simple precautions, you can ensure you don't injure yourself while stretching or cause any pain.

There are different yoga poses you can include in your exercise of mindful stretching. In fact, most of the yoga poses include some form of stretching.

Body Scan

To start this exercise, you can either lie horizontally on the ground with your face and torso facing upward or sit on a chair. If you are sitting on a chair, ensure that your feet are planted firmly on the ground while your hands lie on your thighs. Choose a comfortable position to start the exercise.

Allow your concentration to focus solely on your body, and avoid fidgeting or moving around during this exercise. Only make deliberate movements when you have to readjust your position.

This technique primarily uses your breath to create a center of awareness. Use your breath to concentrate on your body. Don't try to change the way you breathe; once you become aware of your breathing, the next step is to pay attention to your body. Observe how you feel within your skin and observe the way your body feels. Notice how the surface you are lying on (or sitting on) feels, your surroundings, and your body temperature. While doing this, become more conscious and aware of any pain, soreness, tiredness, or tingling sensations in different parts of your body. Also, make a mental note of different parts of your body where you don't feel any sensation or are extremely sensitive.

While performing a body scan, you need to concentrate on every single part of your body, from the tips of your toes to the crown of your head. Don't ignore anything. Slowly shift your focus from one part of the body to another and take note of how you feel.

Once you have taken stock of every single part of your body, it is time to end the body scan. To do this, slowly bring your awareness back to your surroundings. Shift your focus to your breathing by concentrating on the way breath enters and leaves your body. It is time to slowly open your eyes and get back to the real world.

Daily Mindfulness

MBCT prescribes different techniques of mindfulness you can perform in your everyday life. These activities help make you more aware of your body, mind, and any emotions or feelings you experience. Once you become aware of all these things, it becomes easier to change any undesirable beliefs or emotions. Mindfulness can be practiced while showering, eating, exercising, washing dishes, even while making your bed in the morning.

As mindfulness requires a lot of practice, practicing everyday mindfulness is the best way to teach it as a lifestyle. Taking the opportunity to practice mindfulness whenever you are presented with it will help you maintain a healthy sense of awareness and balance throughout your day. This is seen in:

Mindful showering, which is about keeping your attention on just what you can see, hear, feel as you take your shower. While showering, most of us tend to think about different things. Avoid doing this. Concentrate only on the way the water feels on your body. Imagine that the water is washing away all your stress and anxieties — concentrate on cleansing your physical body, and nothing else. Pay attention to the temperature of the water, the way soap feels on your body or any other sensation you experience while lathering yourself.

Mindful eating is keeping your attention on whatever it is you are eating. Whenever you are eating, ensure that your entire concentration is on the meal you consume. Get rid of any electronics or other distractions, which will allow you to focus on the task of eating. Slowly chew your food before you swallow it. Learn to savor every morsel you eat. It is a great way to become more aware of the kind of food you feed your body.

Mindful dishwashing should only be done when you have a few dishes to wash. Mindful dishwashing is watching yourself clean the dirty dishes and listening to the sounds of dishwashing, such as water flowing. You can even pay attention to the smells if you are okay with that.

Mindfully making your bed is done by moving deliberately and with purpose while making your bed. Try to make your bed carefully and deliberately. If you usually are quite quick and careless while doing this, start paying attention to the task at hand. Even if it is a rather mundane activity, it is a great way to bring awareness to yourself. Concentrate on the texture of the sheets, the softness of the mattress, or even the way the pillows look. Put your all into what you are doing, as uninteresting as it may seem.

Pay attention to your muscle tone, your breathing patterns, and your gait. We tend to get trapped in the distractions of heavy breathing and pain during exercise; try to give yourself an experience without all these. Practicing daily mindfulness is an opportunity to maintain awareness and create balance throughout your day.

It is quite important to spend time with your loved ones, but you also need a little time for yourself. Take a break from everything and spend some time with yourself. During the "me" time, avoid any distractions; keep your phone away, don't check your emails or watch TV. There is time to get back to these tasks later. For now, concentrate on how your body feels, your thoughts, and any emotions you are experiencing. Forget about the external world and tune into yourself. It is a great way to practice self-love. Once you become aware of all this, it becomes easier to heal your body.

Mindful observation is a simple exercise that enables you to connect with everything going on in your surroundings. Most of us are often in a hurry, and we miss out on the little things in life. Start by choosing an object present in your immediate surroundings and focus only on that object for a couple of minutes. You can concentrate on a flower, tree, cloud, or anything else that you want. While doing this, carefully observe everything about the object. Once you feel calmer and no thoughts are running wild in your head, it is time to get back to your normal life.

Mindful awareness helps increase your awareness as well as build an appreciation for all the routine activities you perform. Think of any activity you perform several times daily. Perhaps it could be opening a door, drinking water, or anything else that you might have simply taken for granted. Stop for a moment and think about how you feel whenever you perform the activity. How do you feel when you are drinking water? How do you feel when you switch on your laptop? The next time you come across something that makes you smile, learn to appreciate it. It could be something as simple as sharing a meal with your loved ones or having a comfortable bed in which to sleep at night. Instead of going through your life on autopilot, take a couple of minutes to appreciate all the good in your life.

Mindful listening is the ability to listen without any judgment or bias. Our reactions, perceptions, and thoughts about most things that we see and hear daily are all based on our past experiences. Once you learn the skill of mindful listening, you can listen to everything you come across from a neutral perspective. You can start with something as simple as listening to songs. Don't judge a song based on its lyrics, genre, artist, title, or anything else. Instead, simply listen to it and allow your mind to explore the music. Allow yourself to get lost in the rhythm and sound. The idea is to let go of any preconceived notions and try to get involved in the present.

Mindful immersion helps create contentment in the present. It is about living through a routine instead of just getting things done before you move onto something else. Don't think of decluttering as a tiresome chore, and instead pay attention to all the little details that go into this activity. The aim is to try and find new emotions while performing repetitive tasks. When you become aware of all the things that you do, your willingness to do them increases while elevating your overall experience.

Mindful appreciation is quite straight forward. Take a couple of minutes daily and notice any five things you haven't appreciated in your daily life. This exercise helps you become more appreciative of all the seemingly insignificant things in your life. Most of us forget about all the little things in life because we are concentrated on attaining the goals. Learn to be grateful for every single aspect of your life. You probably have things that you wished for a couple of years ago. So, why don't you be grateful for all that you have now? Instead of being filled with regret later, it is better to be a little appreciative right now.

Avoid being judgmental. Mindfulness is your ability to accept everything about yourself. Accept the feelings, thoughts, and sensations you experience. Even all those things that you might have labeled as dangerous and self-destructive are still a part of you. Instead of ignoring them or stuffing them away in a dark corner of your mind, accept them. Merely accepting these things will not make them come true. Learn to understand that your thoughts are just thoughts. Unless you act on them, they will not become real. So, don't allow yourself to be overburdened by all this. Once you let go of all this, you will feel better about yourself. All the stress you used to experience will slowly melt away.

Regardless of the task, you are performing, ensure that all your attention is focused on the task at hand and nothing else. By doing this, you will not only be able to give 100% to the activities you are engaged in, but also improve your self-awareness. If you want to increase your efficiency as well as effectiveness, then start being mindful daily.

Other Meditative Practices

Other meditative practices generally involve two basic categories of focus: the concentrative and the non-concentrative. The concentrative speaks to having a particular object in the center, such as a candle flame, while the non-concentrative has a broader focus, such as the sounds in your environment. Note, however, that some of these focuses do have an overlapping of categories. Below is a short description of some of these practices:

Basic Meditation

Meditation involves sitting in a relaxed position purging your mind or concentrating your psyche on nothing.

Focused Meditation

This is just the primary type but you have something you are focusing on, though you are not to engage your thoughts or attention on it.

Spiritual Meditation

Though meditation is not specific to any one religion, it can be a spiritual practice. Prayer to seek guidance or inner wisdom can be a form of meditation to many people.

Things to Keep in Mind as You Meditate

• Consistent practice matters more than long inconsistent practice, but to get the best results, having a short daily practice with an occasional long exercise such as going to a mindfulness retreat is advisable.

• Regular practice matters more than a perfect method, as any meditation is better than none. So do not waste time trying to figure out the details of the technique; start! Everything else will fall into place.

• Accept that it is normal for your mind to wander even when meditating.

To conclude, don't wait any longer – get into a comfortable sitting posture and start meditating!

Chapter Ten: Don't Panic! How to Stop a Panic Attack with Mindfulness

Panic attacks are sudden, severe surges of fear, panic, and anxiety; they are overwhelming, and people with a panic attack can show both physical as well as emotional symptoms. It involves sudden feelings of terror that strike without warning, and it can occur at any time, even during sleep. Panic attacks might make you think you are dying, going crazy, or having a heart attack. However, this might not be real; the fear and terror may be unrelated to what is happening around you and not be in proportion to the actual situation.

Signs and Symptoms

Panic attacks present with symptoms such as difficulty in breathing, quivering, profuse sweating, and a throbbing pulse. In other cases, you may experience chest pain, or feel detached from yourself.

Panic attacks may occur when you are calm or anxious. Although the panic attack is a symptom of panic disorder, it is normal to have panic attacks in the context of other psychological disorders. For example, if you have a social anxiety disorder, you might have a panic attack before giving a speech at a conference. If you have an obsessive-compulsive disorder, you might have a panic attack when prevented from engaging in a ritual. Panic attacks are not pleasant and can affect social behavior.

Panic attacks are the onset of severe fear or discomfort that reaches the highest point within minutes. You can know if you're having a panic attack if you have at least four of the symptoms below:

· Shortness of breath.

· A feeling of being choked.

· Pain in the chest region.

· Unsteadiness and nausea.

· A pounding heart, clear palpitation, or an accelerated heart rate.

· Trembling or shaking, and sweating.

· Abdominal problems.

· Dizziness, feeling light-headed or faint.

· Paresthesia (numbness or tingling sensations).

· Feelings of being detached from reality or yourself.

· Chills.

· Being afraid of losing yourself.

Panic Attack Versus Panic Disorder

Having a panic attack doesn't necessarily mean that you have a panic disorder; they are quite different. One in three adults will experience at least one panic attack in their lifetime, but most of them will not have panic disorder.

A panic attack can come from being stressed. A few other diseases such as phobias or post-traumatic stress disorder can also present with the symptom of panic attacks. For example, in post-traumatic stress disorder, a panic attack can happen when a person goes back to the place the trauma occurred. These people are usually scared of their shock and not of the panic attack itself.

How to Know if you have Panic Disorder

There are several ways to help you figure out if you actually have a panic disorder and are not simply experiencing a panic attack. Some of these include:

- If it happens a lot.

- If you are prone to experiencing a lot of fear of having another attack.

- If it usually comes on unexpectedly.

- If you find yourself sitting near exits or bathrooms, so you have an easy escape route in case you get an attack.

- If you are scared that certain bad things might happen if you get an attack, like being embarrassed in public.

- If you avoid specific locations or situations and only allow yourself to experience them if you have a friend or family member with you or certain items like medications.

- If you are avoiding physical activities, food, or day-to-day activities because you fear they might trigger a panic attack.

- If you have any one or more of these, then it would be a good idea to see a doctor.

Anxiety Attack Versus Panic Attack

Most people use the terms anxiety and panic attack interchangeably, but they are two different experiences. The DSM-5 describes the features of panic disorder or panic attacks that occur due to another mental disorder. Panic attacks begin to subside after reaching their peak level of intensity at about 10 minutes. In contrast, anxiety is used to describe a core feature of multiple different anxiety disorders. The symptoms that result from being in a state of stress (such as restlessness, shortness of breath, increased heart rate, and difficulty in concentrating) may feel like an attack but are not generally as intense as those experienced at the height of a panic attack.

Who it Affects

Panic attack or disorder can affect anyone, but there are certain groups of people that it affects more often than others.

- Females: like most other anxiety disorders, mature females are more likely to experience a panic attack or disorder than grown males.

- Adults: panic disorder often appears in mid-twenties, although it can happen at any age. Most people with a panic disorder experienced the onset before the age of 33. Though it can exist in kids, it's often not noticed until they are matured.

- People who are suffering from chronic illness: most people with panic attacks or disorder report having at least one other diagnosed chronic physical or mental illness.

- You are at a higher risk of having a panic disorder if you have a family history of such.

Causes

People with specific genes are susceptible to panic disorder. However, the particular genetic patterns associated with high susceptibility have not been identified. You are at a higher risk of developing panic attacks if either or both of your parents have been diagnosed with depression, anxiety, or bipolar disorder.

Panic attacks can be triggered by:

- Work stress
- Social stress

- Various phobias

- Withdrawal from drugs or alcohol

- Chronic conditions or pain

- Medications or supplements

- Driving

- Caffeine

- Memories of severe trauma that happened in the past

Duration of a Panic Attack

Although the time varies between individuals, panic attacks typically reach their highest point within ten minutes or more, and then symptoms begin to decline. Panic attacks seldom last for more than an hour, with most lasting for around thirty minutes.

How often does a panic attack happen?

It is different for different people, you might have one panic attack and never experience another, and you might have attacks once a month or even several times a week.

Can a panic attack kill you?

Panic attacks cause different issues, and many people feel they are about to die when they experience it. However, having a panic attack cannot kill you.

Ways to Stop a Panic Attack

Mindfulness is related closely to meditation and can be practiced at any time, whether you are walking, taking a rest, or working out. Mindfulness is like meditation in motion. Mindful people are optimistic about the present, and they keep an open mind. They are not contemplating or giving a thought to things of the past, nor are they worried about what the future holds. Mindfulness requires that you keep a mind without worries. You will need to gather your focus and perception from inside your head to outside your head because there are a lot of more exciting things on the outside. You can practice mindfulness while walking and working outdoors and during sports. It is mindfulness that will help you shift your attention away from the pain endured during exercise to having a pleasant sensation. Mindfulness will change your perspective of whatever situation you apply it to, and consistent practice of mindfulness will eventually improve your thought patterns and your general mindset.

Here are a few steps to stop a panic attack:

- Breathe deeply.
- Recognize it as a panic attack.
- Close your eyes.
- Practice mindfulness.
- Focus on an object.
- Relax your muscles.
- Find your happy place.
- Engage in light exercise.
- Repeat your mantra.
- Take benzodiazepines.

Recognize that it's a panic attack and not a heart attack

Panic attacks come with the symptom of thinking there is a danger ahead of you or that you are dying. These symptoms can be scary, but the first thing to do is to take away this fear and acknowledge that you are merely having a panic attack. Ascertain that there is no impending doom and remind yourself that this is temporary, it will pass, and you will be okay. This acceptance will allow you to focus on other techniques to treat your symptoms.

Deep breathing

The first practical way to deal with a panic attack is to practice deep breathing. Focus on breathing in deeply and slowly through the nose until the air fills your chest, then sigh out through your mouth. After every few breaths, you should relax to regain your rhythm. The essence of deep breathing is controlled breathing. It is vital you take note of the counts for optimum breathing and to prevent hyperventilation. Hyperventilation can worsen other symptoms; however, if you can control your breath with the counts, you are less likely to experience this.

Shut out any visual stimuli

A loud environment, with various visual stimuli, can trigger your panic attack. Once you feel you have a panic attack, closing your eyes will reduce these stimuli and prevent taking in more visual information so you can easily focus on breathing and controlling the attack.

Focus object

Focusing on a single object can be beneficial during a panic attack. Look for an object that is close to you and carefully analyze it. Trying to explain it will shift your mind to the object and take your mind off other symptoms of the panic attack. For instance, you may choose to analyze how a shoe is placed in its rack carefully. If it's improperly placed or doesn't fit in, you can try describing how it should be to yourself, or what kind of shoe would fit in its place. With this quick focus, whatever panic symptoms you are feeling may subside.

Mindfulness

A panic attack can quickly get you detached from reality. Keeping your mind in the present can redirect your senses away from the intensity of the anxiety. You can give yourself a little task. Identify four things that are around you, feel the texture of three objects, listen to two different sounds, or smell something that can trigger a memory. This exercise aims to keep you grounded in reality and not moving from one worry to another.

Muscle relaxation techniques

A popular technique for coping with panic attacks is muscle relaxation. Sometimes your muscles may become tense unconsciously in response to what you feel to be a dangerous situation. Muscle relaxation techniques help you to control your body's response. In this technique, you repeatedly flex your muscles and then relax them. After the relaxation, you should remain seated to allow yourself to become alert again. This technique is most effective when you have practiced it before a panic attack occurs.

Happy place

You probably have a place or a view that makes you feel utterly relaxed. When you have a panic attack, you can close your eyes and picture yourself in your happy place. You can create a mental picture of the beautiful view that got to you when you were on the plane, or the tranquility you get any time you are listening to music at the beach. However, try not to think of noisy areas like a busy park or a crowded street, even if these are places you enjoy in your everyday life.

The internal mantra

Ever seen someone about to have a panic attack just close their eyes and start moving their lips? Most likely, they're repeating a phrase or two in their head that helps them deal with the attack. Repetition of a mantra, even without speaking it aloud, can be relaxing, and it gives you something to hold on to during a panic attack. Find one that clicks with you and that you can easily remember; repeat it continuously until you feel the panic attack starting to dissipate.

Light exercise

Endorphins are a lifesaver. When our brain releases this chemical into our blood stream we feel happy and energized. Light exercise does wonders when it comes to flooding our system with endorphins, and this ultimately improves our mood drastically. You can choose a light workout that is gentle on the body when you are stressed, like taking a stroll or maybe a quick jog around the park.

Benzodiazepines

Although benzodiazepines can be addictive, they are a medication that may help you treat panic attacks. Just remember that the body can easily adjust to it over time, and it should therefore only be used on rare occasions and in cases of pressing need. When you are having serious panic attacks and can feel one coming on in the worst of situations, that's when this will come in handy.

Keep a diary

Keeping a note of what happens every time you get anxious or have a panic attack can help you spot patterns in what triggers these experiences for you, and this will, in turn, help you to think about how to deal with these situations in the future. You can also try keeping a note of times when you can manage your anxiety successfully; this can, in turn, help you feel more in control of the stress you feel.

How to Help Someone with a Panic Attack

If you ever encounter a person suffering from a panic attack, do not fear. You should not add to the person's stress by panicking or shouting at them. Instead, you can try some of these ways to help.

- Stay calm, do not scream or add your fear to the person's distress.

- Ask questions. If it's not their first time, ask if they use certain medications and if you can help them with it.

- Don't think you know everything that is going on. Ask them the cause of the panic and what they need.

- Be encouraging and positive while talking to them in simple sentences they can easily understand.

- Prevent the person from going into hyperventilation by encouraging them to breathe more slowly and deeply.

You can also say to the person things like:

- "What can I do to help you get through this?"

- "You are doing fine, and I am proud of you."

- "This attack is not dangerous at all, although it might feel scary."

Take this simple approach, and you will find out that you can:

- Reduce the amount of stress in a very stressful situation.

- Prevent the worse from happening in the situation.

- Curb a complicated experience.

You can help someone recovering from a panic attack by:

- Giving the person the autonomy to proceed in therapy at his or her own pace.

- Being patient and addressing all efforts toward recovery, though the person may not meet all of the goals.

- Avoiding things or situations that can cause anxiety.

- Not panicking, even when the other person panics.

It is all right to be concerned and anxious yourself, but you can control yourself and the situation.

Fortunately, panic disorder and panic attack is a treatable condition, even to the extent of complete disappearance. Psychotherapy and medications have been used as effective treatments, either singly or combined. If another medication is necessary, your doctor may prescribe medicines for anxiety. There are certain antidepressants or anticonvulsant drugs that also have anti-anxiety properties, and a type of heart medication known as beta-blockers, which help to prevent and control the episodes of panic disorder.

Chapter Eleven: How to Prevent a Relapse

Lapse: A lapse is a brief return to feeling down or to your old habits. It is a common and temporary situation.

Relapse: As opposed to a lapse, a relapse is a complete deterioration or complete return to your initial state of health after a temporary improvement.

For example, you had a phobia of spiders, and now you know that it is best not to scream when seeing one. Somewhat, you calm yourself down, breathe, tell yourself some coping thoughts, and gradually ignore the spider. So, if you find a spider in your room one day and you scream, that is a lapse. If you then go back to screaming and running whenever you see a spider, then we can call that a relapse.

Lapses can progress to relapses, but this should not necessarily happen. You can stop a lapse from escalating into a relapse.

When Does a Lapse Become a Relapse?

The general belief that what you say to yourself after a failure can make or break you is very much applicable here. What you think and say to yourself after a lapse can lead you back to the right track or throw you into relapse. Seeing a lapse as a failure can keep you sick and lead to a relapse. A better perspective is that you were able to have emotional wellness before, you can have it again; process whatever happened before and learn from your mistake.

Going back to our spider-phobia example: if, after avoiding the spider all day, you said to yourself, "It looks like I'm bringing back old habits; I need to do better tomorrow and get myself together!" you would discover that your lapse would probably decline or stop completely, and now you can face your anxieties and fears head on. If you avoided spiders all day, and at the end of the day said to yourself, "All my hard work is a waste, now I'm here again. Arggghhh, I'm such a jerk! Why am I even trying when there is no cure?" This is not really helpful, and it won't help your recovery.

Can I Prevent Lapses and Relapses?

Yes, you can prevent lapses and relapses, and here are seven clues you can use:

Do not give up on practicing; the best way to prevent a lapse is regularly practicing your CBT skills. If you are practice regularly, you will be in good shape to handle whatever situations you might face.

Understand yourself (Red Flags). Relapse doesn't happen suddenly. It occurs over a period of time. Preventing relapse by understanding yourself is not complicated. Understand yourself by identifying your triggers, asking for help, and sharing your feelings.

New challenges. Everyone is a work in progress, and you are no exception. This means there is always a chance to get better, and you can work on yourself and live a more fulfilling life. It will be less easy to backslide into your old ways if you deliberately work on new ways of overcoming your anxiety. An excellent way to prevent lapses is by challenging yourself regularly and taking up new scary situations. Make a list of cases that sound scary to you and initiate anxiety when you think of them, and work on them.

Learn from Your Past Experiences. Lapses are not synonymous with failure, rather they are opportunities to learn and get better. Figure out the situation that always leads to you having a lapse and make a plan that will help you deal with these situations better in the future.

As said earlier, what you say to yourself after a lapse can impact your behavior. Have a few positive things that you say to yourself. CBT has helped you, and you cannot throw away everything you have learned. Going back to the beginning means having anxiety and not knowing how to handle it. Going back to practicing your CBT skills will help you to master your anxiety again in a short time.

Be kind to yourself; remember that lapses are not the end of your world, take it easy on yourself and learn. No one is above making mistakes; we all make mistakes. We all try to speak nicely to people, so do the same to yourself; don't say harsh things to yourself. Lapses can be a blessing in disguise at times because you get a chance to learn that you can go back to fashion out a new formula of dealing with your situation.

Enjoy yourself; make sure you always take the time to rest and relax from all the hard work you are doing. Appreciate yourself; buy yourself a nice meal, get something new, or hang out with your friends. You can also reward yourself by pampering yourself and taking some time to relax.

Depression Triggers

People who have a history of depression can have triggers that cause a depressive episode. However, an event being stressful for a person does not mean it will trigger depression. Triggers vary from one person to another; what is difficult and stressful for you might be easy for others.

Potential Depression Triggers Include:

Sad occurrences

Various life situations, such as the death of a loved one or a tragic end to a treasured relationship, can be a trigger for depression. According to a study, 20% of people enter into depression after this type of loss.

Stopping Treatment

Most people stray away from treatment after they feel their symptoms are getting better. A high percentage of these people gradually see their symptoms setting in again, and they may enter into another episode of depression. Finishing your treatment can surprisingly lower your risk of relapse.

Traumatic events

Remembering events that have caused trauma in the past can bring about a relapse. People who have had depression resulting from attacks or disasters are at a high risk of entering another episode.

Health Conditions

People who have been diagnosed with particular health conditions can lose their self-esteem and confidence. They may enter into overthinking and, consequently, into depression. If you find yourself in this category, take care of your medical condition and prevent it from taking over your life. This will give you control over the depression.

Financial issues

Money problems are prevalent causes of worry. A way to avoid this is to practice a healthy economic lifestyle. Create a budget and stay true to the budget. Also, you might want to create a savings plan, so you are not tempted to spend all your money at once. Attend programs that don't cost a fortune so that you can spend time with family and friends. Increased financial stability can reduce your risk of having a relapse.

Other factors you need to identify and avoid include:

· Hormone changes

· Addictive behaviors

· Sexual problems

· Poor sleep habits and diets

· Feeling stressed and overwhelmed

Ways to Minimize Depression Triggers

Not all depression triggers are inescapable; some can be avoided.

It is best you learn how to find your way around these triggers as much as you can. If you are starting to get overwhelmed, here are some steps that can help you out:

Stay Positive

Find ways to improve your self-esteem, and regularly say encouraging words to yourself.

Be social

Relate with friends, family, and reach out to them when you begin to feel your symptoms getting overwhelming.

Avoid Alcohol

There is a false belief that alcohol makes you feel better; though it may seem like it, the truth is that it can make your depression worse.

Early Signs of a Depression Relapse

If you've had a history of depression, symptoms might start appearing again and trigger worry; this is totally understandable. People who have experienced depression before may have a recurrence after a period of time. This period can range from weeks to years, sometimes many years after the occurrence. If you can spot the red flags early, you might be able to stop severe episodes from occurring.

About half of the people who overcome an episode of depression for the first time will remain well. For others, depression can come back a few times throughout their lives. People have different degrees of recurrence; some experience sadness or just want to avoid daily activities. However, if you have these feelings almost daily for more than two weeks, and it begins to affect work or social life, then you may be experiencing depression.

Two ways depression can return are:

When symptoms start to appear again or worsen during recovery from an earlier episode, we can say relapse is looming. Relapse is likely to occur within two months of stopping treatment.

Most recurrence occurs within the first six months after recovery from the previous episodes.

Around 20% of people usually experience a recurrence, but this can rise when depression is severe.

We have some depression-like disorders that can return frequently. These include:

Seasonal affective disorder (SAD): SAD occurs mostly during the winter months, due to the decrease in sunlight.

Premenstrual dysphoria syndrome (PDS): PDS is a severe form of premenstrual syndrome.

Early Signs of Depression Relapse

Some people have their depression symptoms occur once; for others, it can occur over and over. It is essential to pay attention to your symptoms when they occur because this will quickly help you catch a possible sign of relapse. Early signs that you might have a relapse include;

· Having extremes of sleeping disorders; excessive sleep or lack of sleep

· Loss of interest in activities you enjoyed doing before

· A depressed feeling of sadness and anxiousness

· Memory issues

· Feeling regrets over past events

· Thoughts of or attempts at suicide

· Avoiding social conversations and relationships with people

· Extremes of appetite leading to excessive weight gain or loss

Suicide Prevention

People who commit suicide must have talked about it once or more in their conversations, no matter how serious it did or did not sound. Do not ignore these signs. Many of these people try to seek help, and they want the pain to stop. Take any suicidal talk seriously and try to yield to their cry for help. Here are a few tips to respond to someone if you notice any signs of suicide.

· Listen to their conversations honestly, and if you're unsure if they are suicidal, ask nicely.

· Respond quickly to severe suicidal risk. Put a call through a local crisis center, call 911, remove harmful objects from the area, and do not leave them alone.

· Get professional care and follow-up treatment.

If you are having suicidal thoughts, don't use suicidal talks to give someone an idea that you are thinking about suicide. Instead, open up honestly, and you can save a life.

Tips for Preventing a Relapse

People suffering from episodes of depression can have crushing, intense feelings. The following strategies can help prevent depression relapse:

· Have supporting relationships.

· Avoid isolation. It is imperative to surround yourself with understanding, kind, and supportive people.

· Avoid and modify depressive thinking patterns.

· CBT can help you change your thinking style. Most people suffering from depression have negative thinking patterns. These patterns can be changed, and CBT techniques we've discussed can be useful for you for a lifetime.

· Follow your prescribed medication.

· Work together with your psychiatrist and follow any treatment pattern they give you.

· Be ready for a relapse. It is advisable to plan for relapse and act upon signs as quickly as they appear.

Correcting and Coping with a Relapse

Having a return to unhelpful anxiety reactions and old thought patterns might mean that the initial treatment is not working effectively. We recommend that you seek your doctor's advice and preferably change your treatment strategy. Another treatment option is the use of medications like antidepressants or mood stabilizers with the doctor's prescription. If you've been on medication before, and it seems to be failing, you can talk to your doctor about a change in dosage.

Conclusion

The effectiveness of CBT is one of the primary reasons why it is being used all over the world to improve mental health. Long gone are the days when doctors and therapists used to focus solely on drugs and other pharmaceuticals as treatment. CBT can help treat anxiety, personality disorders, depression, and other behavioral problems associated with mental health.

Prioritizing your mental health is as important as taking care of your physical health. A healthy body will not do you much good if your mind is continuously plagued with negativity. You can always seek help and try cognitive behavioral therapy to improve your mental wellbeing. Now that you are armed with all the information you need, it is time to get started as soon as possible!

Thank you and all the best!

References

Ben, M. (2019). In-Depth: Cognitive-behavioral therapy. Retrieved from

https://psychcentral.com/lib/in-depth-cognitive-behavioral-therapy

Rosy B, et al. What to expect in CBT. Retrieved from
http://cogbtherapy.com/what-happens-in-cbt

Mental illness. Retrieved from https://www.mayoclinic.org/diseases-conditions/mental-illness/symptoms-causes/syc-20374968

Diagnostic and Statistical Manual of Mental Disorders DSM-5. 5th ed. Arlington, Va.: American Psychiatric Association; 2013. https://dsm.psychiatryonline.org. Accessed November 2019.

Healthline Editorial team, and medically reviewed by Timothy, J. (2017). Signs of Depression. Retrieved from https://www.healthline.com/health/depression/recognizing-symptoms

Erica, J. (2018). 11 signs and symptoms of anxiety disorders. Retrieved from https://www.healthline.com/nutrition/anxiety-disorder-symptoms#section2

Deanna, R. (2016). How to Create Achievable Goals for Your Mental Wellness. Retrieved from https://www.goodtherapy.org/blog/how-to-create-achievable-goals-for-your-mental-wellness-0822164

Mark, T. (2016). 3 Instantly Calming CBT Techniques for Anxiety: Cognitive-behavioral tools that anyone can use. Retrieved from https://www.unk.com/blog/3-instantly-calming-cbt-techniques-for-anxiety/

Chris, C. Treating depression with Cognitive Behavioral Therapy. Retrieved from https://journeypureriver.com/treating-depression-cognitive-behavioral-therapy/

3 CBT tips to help overcome workplace stress. Retrieved from https://www.efficacy.org.uk/blog/corporate-wellbeing/3-cbt-tips-to-help-overcome-workplace-stress/

Sheri, J. (2014). CBT vs. MBCT – What is the Difference? Retrieved from https://www.harleytherapy.co.uk/counselling/cbt-mbct-difference.htm

Courtney, E. (2019). What are Intrusive Thoughts in OCD & how to get rid of them? Retrieved from https://positivepsychology.com/intrusive-thoughts/

Kimberly, H, and medically reviewed by Timothy J.L (2019). Intrusive Thoughts: Why We Have Them and How to Stop Them. Retrieved from https://www.healthline.com/health/mental-health/intrusive-thoughts#causes

Mindfulness Animated in 3 minutes. Retrieved from AnimateEducate. https://www.youtube.com/watch?v=mjtfyuTTQFY

Katharina, S, and medically reviewed by Steven, G. (2019). Use Mindfulness Meditation to Ease Anxiety. Retrieved from https://www.verywellmind.com/mindfulness-meditation-exercise-for-anxiety-2584081

Ana, G et al. (2018). 11 ways to stop a Panic Attack. Retrieved from https://www.healthline.com/health/how-to-stop-a-panic-attack#recognize-panic-attack

Panic Free TV. Meditation for panic attacks: does mindfulness work? Retrieved from https://www.youtube.com/watch?v=_EbqcVH9eVg

Symptoms of a Panic Attack. Retrieved from Anxiety and Depression Association of America. https://adaa.org/understanding-anxiety/panic-disorder-agoraphobia/symptoms

How to Prevent a Relapse. Retrieved from Anxiety Canada. https://anxietycanada.com/sites/default/files/RelapsePrevention.pdf

Regina, B.W. (2016). 7 Factors That Can Trigger a Depression Relapse. Retrieved from https://www.everydayhealth.com/hs/major-depression-health-well-being/factors-can-trigger-depression-relapse/

Timothy, J. (2019). What are the early signs of a depression relapse? Retrieved from https://www.medicalnewstoday.com/articles/320269.php